The Ultimate Weight Loss Guide for Women of Any Age to Permanently Lose Weight Fast

Discover the Power of Mindset, Meditation, and Different Diet and Exercise Plans To Finally Take Back Control of Your Body Physique

Madison Bright

Table of Contents

Introduction

We've all been there—we have gotten on the scale after weeks of tireless dieting and we see those numbers staring back at us. A sore excuse for "weight loss" if you could even call it that, even though that was the aim and the ultimate goal of the endless salads, the constant cravings, and the relentless hunger.

I know the scale becomes our worst enemy when we are on a journey of bettering ourselves. But let's be honest, the best motivation you'll ever have is seeing the numbers actually decrease. I have found myself in the same position that you may be in right now. I have found myself scouring the web for ways to "lose 10 pounds in two weeks," I have found myself trying and testing every diet under the sun only to be met with disappointment after what was a beautiful Sunday lunch—the joy I felt the day before shamefully melting away into self-loathing as I watched the numbers jump up on that Monday morning. A week of tireless effort and starvation, shattered by the extra slice of French loaf that I thought I could indulge in.

I have also been on the dark end of weight loss. I have been in the position of mercilessly starving myself, on the verge of developing unhealthy eating disorders, just to see some sort of distorted idea of perfection that I had in my mind staring back at me in the mirror. The goals that I had for my body physically seemed almost impossible to achieve. I have even gotten to the point of negative self-talk where I told myself that I don't care how unhealthy I am; as long as I lose some weight, I will be happy.

But this happiness, this false idea that my mind wickedly created knowing full well it couldn't be achieved, dangled in front of me, the carrot laughing at the donkey who was ultimately destined to fail.

And that is when I realized that my entire mentality and my entire approach to this endeavor were completely wrong, distorted, and warped by none other than myself.

You see, my false expectations for my own body made these goals that I set for myself unrealistic and unachievable. I was setting myself up for disappointment. No matter how hard I worked, neither genetics, my frame, nor my body that birthed two kids would have been able to reach the goal I set for myself. It was then that I realized that weight loss isn't just about shredding the extra pounds from around my waist. Instead, it was about changing my lifestyle, and more importantly, it was about becoming healthy.

What good was losing 20 lbs. if it was going to weaken all the muscles in my body, including my heart? What good was weight loss and having a bikini body if I was too weak and malnourished to even head to the beach?

My mind completely changed in the way I approached weight loss and the way I approached my health, which I realized was a fundamental component that needs to be considered throughout the weight loss journey.

Since making a lifestyle change, and making a long-term promise to my body, I have found a new vigor for life. I have consistently trained and have found my comfort in eating the right foods for my body type. Since endeavoring on my own journey, I have helped many of my own friends on their weight loss journey. And now, I have decided to help others better achieve their weight loss and health goals.

What This Book Is About

Gone are the days when you would be searching the internet for the next quick-fix diet that promises unrealistic amounts of weight loss in unrealistic time frames. Gone are your days of trying diet fad after diet fad only to go back to your old version of normal and have the weight pile back on. Gone are the days of spending your hard-earned money on weight loss books that either tell you what you already know or make no significant contribution to your health without coercing you into purchasing unnecessary subscriptions.

This is your permanent solution to weight loss and to health.

This book does not make a promise to you that you will lose a specific number of pounds in a certain number of days. Let's be honest, those promises might be fake, and whether it is because I am lying or because you are sneaking candy bars in after everyone has gone to bed, a one-size-fits-all approach is guaranteed to never work. Instead, this book is going to help you learn your body, not just at this stage in life, but every other stage that is to come. This book is going to help you make a promise to yourself and your body that everything you do will be for the benefit of this one and only body you have.

I am here to help you, the extraordinary and beautiful woman reading this book. I am here to help you take back control of your life, your body, and your physique. I am here to help you feel more confident and feel more positive about yourself and how you look.

Losing weight is not just about eating less. Instead, it is about mindset and discipline; it is about meditation; it is about finding a long-term eating plan that works for your body type, and it is about finding an exercise plan that you can successfully stick to.

At its most fundamental level, ideal and healthy weight loss is about finding balance. It is not only about the physical part of life but also the mental and emotional aspects of life. For that reason, we are also going to delve into the psychology of weight loss and research that has been conducted on these components. We need to factor in genetics, and why your body is shaped the way it is (you wouldn't hope to be 6'2" when your entire family is under 5'5"). We will look at meditation practices that align your body with your mind, and we will look at ways that fasting can in some ways add to weight loss and in other ways take away from weight loss.

No matter what age you are, you can achieve the desired confidence you may have always lacked. Let us go on a journey of finding a body that you feel confident in and feel 100% and truly yourself in. You will easily fit into the physique that makes you feel like you can do anything.

Are you going to love every second of it? Probably not. Will you fall in love with every other aspect of life so much more? Definitely. The only way for this weight loss change to be permanent is if you make a forever promise to your body and make a commitment to a lifestyle change. You can't diet forever, but you can strike a healthy balance forever.

So come with me on this journey and allow me to introduce you to the new you; the you who is confident, beautiful, and most importantly, who loves the skin she is in. You are going to love her!

Chapter 1:

The True Meaning of Weight Loss

Let me tell you a secret: Weight loss cannot be successfully achieved just by reducing what you eat. This may come as a surprise to you, or it may have been something you knew all along, but sources of false information get many people to starve themselves in an attempt to lose weight.

Now, if you have been one of those people, you may have found yourself feeling weak, frustrated, tired, and just downright hangry. That is because your body is not meant to live in survival mode, eating meals that are sparsely spread apart. Now, while you may have heard the words "calorie deficit" thrown around a lot on your weight loss journey, what people fail to explain to tell you is how to achieve the perfect balance of a calorie deficit. You see, a calorie deficit means eating less than the metabolic energy your body uses for breathing, keeping your heart beating, digesting, and everything else that your body does in a day just to keep itself alive. But a calorie deficit needs to be within specific and healthy ranges for your body to realize that it can lose the weight without it going into shock and fear, holding onto every ounce of food in fear that it may never gain nourishment again.

But before we can even look at eating habits, physical activity, and lifestyle change, we need to back up and start at the beginning, unlike many of the diet plans which throw you into an eating plan that doesn't match your body type or your lifestyle.

Knowing Your Physique

One thing I have learned through my time in health and fitness is that no two bodies are the same. Yes, you have heard this many times before, but how many times have you, someone who rarely engages in physical activity, looked at an Instagram fitness influencer and desired to have the exact same body that they have? Why wouldn't you want that? Their flat tummy has cuts and creases in all the right places, and they only ever seem to own bikinis and crop tops; but if you are being honest, if your body looked like that, you also wouldn't wear anything else either. This becomes your goal, and this is what you aspire to work toward. But what you don't realize is that you are the one setting your own self up for failure. Your 5'2" body frame with broad hips will never look like the 6'1" Instagram model. This is because we all have different physiques, and the best way to set a goal and achieve that physique is to know and understand your body and make lifestyle changes accordingly.

It is important to realize how healthy a good physique can be, but when I say good physique. I don't mean that someone else's is better than yours, I mean having a good physique on your own unique health spectrum. Having a good physique presents you with a number of beneficial physical and health attributes. At face value, you will look better, feel better, and be able to fit into the clothes you desire. But from a health perspective, it makes your heart stronger by removing the strain that additional fat may be placing on it, you can reduce your cholesterol, blood sugar, and blood pressure, and you can actually add a couple of years onto your life (healthy years, not wheelchair-bound years).

Now, you may be seeing me throw the word "health" around quite a bit, and you are probably thinking that you want to lose weight, but you don't really care about health. But when you shift your focus from weight loss to increased health, weight loss becomes a by-product that follows suit.

Let us first understand the importance of good health. Being healthy gives you power over your body and power over the circumstances that surround your body. But what is good health? Basically, health refers to the physical, mental, and social well-being of an individual and it refers to a person's personal capacities or what they are able to do. It is a tool rather than an objective. For example, if you are not in good mental health, you may not be able to meet the objective of successfully carrying out your work. This may then affect your financial health.

There are different types of health and different factors and variables at play that affect your health in a positive or negative way. Basically, you need good health to achieve societal goals and objectives and to successfully fulfill the functions of being an active member of society. An example would be fulfilling your work duties, playing with your kids, spending time with your family, and much more. And therein lies the importance of good health. You need to be in good mental, physical, and emotional health to do what's important in life.

But this is also why "good health" or the concept and idea behind health is so complex. Since it is not a goal, but rather a tool, it is not something that can be met or achieved. This means that you would be constantly working to maintain good health to achieve other goals. When you consider it this way, it makes sense why weight loss and being healthy is a lifelong commitment to yourself and not a weight goal that you reach before heading out to McDonald's when you see the desired number on the scale.

With that said, good health can easily be a lifelong commitment that is sometimes not easy to achieve. As mentioned, there are constant variables and factors at play that may contribute to or negatively affect your good health (which will impact the life goals you are hoping to achieve). For example, flu season rolls around, you get sick, and you are unable to get in your daily workout or go on a hike with your group of friends. After the flu passes, you again work on achieving good health so that you can head to the gym to build up your stamina for the hike with your friends (even though this is just one example referring to physical health only).

It is easy to see the importance of maintaining good health for the purpose of actually living your day-to-day life to the fullest, but it is difficult to actually measure good health. Things are much easier to monitor and maintain if a number is attributed to it. When it comes to physical health, one way of monitoring good health is by measuring your body mass index (BMI).

The BMI scale uses a calculation to determine if a person has a healthy body weight. By measuring your weight and height in relation to each other, your BMI can be an indication if you have excess body fat, and it can narrow down the possibility of an individual suffering from further health problems. While it doesn't give a diagnosis, it is a tool that is used as an indicator of whether or not you should start worrying about your health. Now I know you might be thinking that everyone has different body types, so how can a standardized system determine if someone is healthy or not? Well, it is simple. Your BMI is gauged on a range that spans more than 10 kgs or 22 lbs.

To calculate your BMI, you would need to divide your weight in kilograms by the square of your height in meters and you will have a number. If, like me, you are not mathematically inclined, there are a number of automated BMI calculator applications that you can download or BMI calculators that you can use online.

If your BMI falls below 18.5, it means that you are underweight (of which there are various ranges, each with a varying degree of severity). If you have a BMI of between 18.5 and 24.9, it means that you have a normal weight range and that you are within the range of a healthy weight. If your BMI is between 25.0 to 29.9, you are considered overweight, and if it is 30.0 or higher, you are considered obese.

It is easy to see from these broad ranges that accommodations can be made for individuals who have different body types, which is what makes body mass indexing such an effective tool.

With that said, it is great to maintain consistency in your body weight and make sure that it is controlled. Ultimately, you will need to control your body weight to get it within a normal and healthy BMI range, and then you will have to maintain a controlled environment to keep it within that healthy range. When you have your body weight under control, you will find your body automatically doing things to work in optimal functionality. You will have the joys of controlled cholesterol, blood sugar, and blood pressure, but your body will actively work toward combating heart disease, arthritis, diabetes, and even some forms of cancer.

Now that I have hopefully convinced you that being healthy should be your primary focus, let me share with you how you can be healthy.

Finding a way of getting healthy is almost always at odds with some "get thin quick" schemes, which can make it hard for you to discern what is real and what is not. But it is also extremely difficult to actually sift through all the information that is available. There are some common wrongs that you may come across on the internet that I can help put to bed once and for all. This will also help you realize what the misconceptions are and what the truths about weight loss are.

One of the greatest and most common misconceptions that you will come across is that you need to stop eating to lose weight. Now, while we have already mentioned that you need to be in a calorie deficit, many people mistake the term "eating less" for "eating almost nothing at all." So, while websites may be giving the correct advice, people often misinterpret it. This means that they overcompensate and try to eat as little as possible in a day. This is neither realistic nor effective. The reasons are that, first, starvation is not effective in the long run, and this is known as a crash diet. Eventually, your body is going to realize that it is not getting enough food. It doesn't know when you are going to feed it again, so it stores everything you eat as fat. This may lead to you gaining weight or quickly reaching a plateau where you can't lose any more weight.

The next reason why this is ineffective is that you begin craving foods that will get you full fast or that will spike your energy levels and sugar to give your body the much-needed kick it so deeply desires. So, even if you are not eating a lot, or often when you do eat, you eat extremely unhealthy foods.

It is not sustainable to starve yourself because, remember, you are approaching weight loss as a healthy, long-term habit that you hope to adopt. You cannot adopt starving yourself as a healthy habit because your body needs energy for survival. Even if you work at a desk all day and you only type on your keyboard, if that was all you did in a day, you would still be burning energy, albeit a smaller amount.

However, what you will actually find as we journey together toward weight loss and a healthy lifestyle is that eating less actually causes more harm than good. You may be inadvertently causing yourself to become malnourished, and you can quickly start to see the negative effects of this in your hair, nails, teeth, skin, and even with your bones becoming more brittle.

Other misconceptions that you may come across when you are trying to lose weight are that you need to go through extreme exercise programs to even begin seeing any change, that carbs need to be avoided like the plague, that you can take certain foods, and even diet pills to speed up metabolism, that you need to stop snacking to achieve weight loss, that weight loss happens in one go and is a once off deal, that you only need to eat salads or bland foods to lose weight, and my favorite, is that all calories are equal.

The reason why that last point, in particular, is my favorite is that I saw this concept entirely disproved in my own life. When you consider that one cupcake has about the same amount of calories in it as around six apples and that two apples fill your tummy with more than one cupcake, it is clear to see that not all calories are created equally. Also, different foods are processed by our bodies differently. If you eat the same amount of calories in protein as you do in carbs, the way your body processes and breaks each one down is different, and the way those calories are spent by your body is different. Therefore, you will find that eating a certain amount of calories in protein, as opposed to the same amount of calories in carbs, the protein will help you lose weight better than the carbs (Gunnars, 2019).

The reason why these misconceptions prove to be true is that weight loss and weight maintenance are actually all about balance. Weight loss can't be all about what you eat, but with no consideration given to physical activity. Instead, you need to be balanced all around. I'm not just talking about what you eat and what exercise you do, instead, you need to lead a balanced lifestyle, you need to find balance in your physical, mental, and emotional condition, and you need to find balance in your dietary and physical habits. For example, your life can't be all about work and you take absolutely no time to rest and spend with your family. This will lead to mental fatigue which is extremely unhealthy.

Getting Healthy

Now that we know about the great balancing act that weight loss actually is, we can use some tips that are generally considered healthy practices to lose weight. These tips include cutting down on processed carbs, not just doing cardio but also strength training, getting your sleeping habits into shape, working on your mental health, keeping a journal, and being mindful about a lot of your tasks.

There are also specific things that you can do on a regular basis, such as drinking enough water, eating fiber, cooking more often than buying food (this is because you know exactly what is going into your meal), eating from a smaller plate, and being mindful of the foods you purchase which will impact not only your weight loss but your overall health as well.

I have also personally found that planning my meals takes the guesswork out of deciding what to eat. I plan a menu for the entire month before I go grocery shopping, and I usually find that when I know exactly what my family is eating, there is no decision fatigue, which often ends in us buying takeout.

Something that most people tend to overlook, or even entirely forget about when they are counting and monitoring their calorie intake, is the drinks that they put into their bodies. It is great that you had a salad for lunch, but you drank three energy drinks throughout the day that are high in calories because that's exactly what energy is—calories. The same goes for your intake of alcohol. Wine, ciders, beers, and all other alcoholic beverages have calories in them. We often forget to count these. When you realize that alcohol doesn't form a necessity in your life, you quickly discover how easy it is to do without it, and just like that, you cut some major calories out of your day.

Lastly, one of the best ways that you can get healthy is by actually enjoying what you eat. I am not talking about eating lettuce only because, news flash, literally no one in the world likes the taste of lettuce. Instead, I am talking about creating healthy meals that you enjoy eating but that are actually good for you. We have been taught to immediately associate health with salads. But this is a distorted view.

Instead, you can enjoy food, all foods at that, if you do it in the right way.

What This Book Will Cover

Considering that everyone is different, this book is going to help you learn your own body. As women, we often wear many different hats, we have endless responsibilities, and our bodies and ourselves are usually the last things to take care of on that list. This book is going to teach you how making yourself a priority will get you the mind and body you deserve.

You will learn what is healthy and what is not, what works for you and what doesn't. We will cover weight loss from a health perspective, making sure to cover elements of diet, physical fitness, mental health, psychological health, and everything in between.

As much as it has been said that you are what you eat, you are actually much more than that, and every complexity that you comprise needs love, and attention. This book is going to teach you how to do that. Following the instructions in this book, coupled with finding the right dietary plan and learning your own unique body type, will give you a healthier lifestyle, of which weight loss is a great perk.

Choosing what works for you means getting to know your body in the current time and space that it exists in. The old version of you could have done intermittent fasting to lose weight, but after two kids, your metabolism might have slowed down and that won't work anymore. Your body is a dynamic and ever-adapting tool constantly changing to survive in the environment that you present to it. You are not only going to learn the best lifestyle for your current body, but for every future version of you, that is still to come.

Chapter 2:

The Journey Toward a Healthy

Lifestyle and Weight Loss Begins

With the Mind

When I say that your mind is the most powerful tool that you own, you may respond with, "I know, I have heard that a thousand times!" Well, guess what I am going to tell you... *Your mind is the most powerful tool that you own.* What if I told you that your calorie intake could affect your mind? For a second, I want you to think about the way you feel when you are hungry. There are people who get hangry, they get easily frustrated, and they become snappy. It is almost like they are replaced with a version of themselves that doesn't shy away from conflict, despite how timid and calm-natured this person may be on a normal day.

Other people become extremely withdrawn, they become quiet, and they don't really engage much in conversation or interactions. This may seem like small examples, but even in these small examples, it is easy to see how hunger affects your mindset and behavior. Now that we have established a relationship between these two components, we could probably flip it around and say that our innate occurrences can affect our outward behavior. This means that if we have a positive mindset, it could probably affect our eating habits.

This is something that should not be underestimated in weight loss, and that is why this entire chapter is going to be dedicated to finding the right mindset for weight loss and for a healthy lifestyle.

Creating the Right Mindset

When you consider that our mindset and our thought processes have the ability to change so much of our physical lives and our circumstances, it is clear to see that weight loss, while greatly dependent on what we put into our body and the physical activity we do, is extremely dependent on our mindset and our mental health. If you have a negative mindset and you approach every aspect of life with a downward and negative approach, the chances of this negativity manifesting in your physical life are very possible. Whether you gain weight, or your immune system is affected and you get sick more often, you will see your body begin to mimic what is happening in your mind. With the way our bodies and our minds are so intricately woven, studies continue to emphasize the importance of maintaining psychological and mental health because of the effects it has on the body's immune system (Vasile, 2020).

The importance of mindset in weight loss stems from a number of different factors including that if you approach your physical health and weight loss journey with positivity and with a positive mindset, you are more likely to experience successes however small they may be, compared to if you focus solely on the negative side of things. Having a positive mindset is important in your ability to stick to a healthy lifestyle and the results you are likely to see. When you have a positive mindset, you feel good about the changes you are making as opposed to dreading the life you are leading. This means that when you see a small change on the scale, you are able to celebrate it and enjoy the change as opposed to dwelling on how small the change is.

When you have a positive mindset, you are also kinder to yourself. We are human, and slip-ups do happen. Whether you forget to take your vitamins or you have two candy bars instead of one, we are bound to make these errors. Being kind to yourself and having the right mindset makes sure that you treat these slip-ups as just that, as opposed to allowing yourself to be pulled into a downhill spiral. This actually stems from our ability to successfully use positive self-talk. We have all been there—you have just eaten four slices of pizza, and you can barely move because while you were eating, you were throwing back a few glasses of beer or Coca-Cola. You sit there wondering why you had that last slice of pizza almost entirely forgetting about the ice cream you had earlier that day. This leads to you relentlessly berating yourself about how little control you have, taking your frustrations out on yourself, and making yourself feel as horrible emotionally as you do physically.

When you have a positive mindset, you can have positive self-talk which means you aren't punishing yourself for a lapse or a setback but instead you understand that everyone makes mistakes. Eventually, you may even find yourself with such a strong mindset that you don't even give in to the cravings and urges to binge eat.

With the right mindset, you have greater control over the types of food you eat and the quality of food you consume. Your mind gets to the point where it serves as a gatekeeper, allowing only the best into your body.

While the importance and the impact of your mindset on your health and your weight loss journey are important, it may seem daunting to establish this positive mindset. Yes, in the beginning, it may be hard, but you would be surprised how easy it actually is, and you would be even more surprised at the positive impact it has on your body.

But how do you cultivate this positive mindset? The reality is that losing weight is hard. The fact that you are here, reading this book, probably means that you have tried many other options and they haven't worked for you, whether it is because the diet itself was flawed, or because your mindset was ready for that change. With that being said, the starting point for any weight loss journey is getting your mindset focused on your goal. At the moment, your mind is pretty much adjusted to where your body is and how it functions in the space around it. Your mind knows which spaces your body is more likely to fit through and what size clothing would be comfortable for you. Whether you avoid shopping altogether or whether you buy two sizes bigger anyway, your mind is comfortable with where it is. We're going to change that.

There is no step-by-step guide that you can follow to change your mindset, but instead, there are things that you need to do consistently to achieve your desired outcome. This means that the tips below can be done in order, but each point needs to be something you continuously work toward and that you constantly remind yourself of each day.

- You need to unlearn everything that you may have learned in the past. This means that you have probably experienced failure in your diets before and that is ultimately the reason why you are looking for a long-term solution. But when so many diets have failed in the past, you may have created and grown accustomed to a failure mindset. This is what you need to unlearn. You need to unlearn that weight loss guides and strategies are ineffectual and cost money because you have to buy supplements because that means you are already approaching any new weight loss approach with negativity. You need to unlearn these flawed patterns. You also need to unlearn the bad habits that you may have picked up in the past when you tried to lose weight. Starving yourself, depriving yourself of variety in the hopes that you lose weight quickly, cutting out meals, and obsessing about the small things are all behaviors that need to be unlearned. This essentially is you setting yourself up for failure and because you are approaching your weight loss with a negative mindset, you basically allow this self-fulfilling prophecy of failure to come true (Fields, 2020). The way to change this is by establishing a positive self-fulfilling prophecy, even if it seems silly at first. Tell yourself that you are going to be a thinner, healthier version of yourself and that you are going to eat healthier. Just like that, you have changed the narrative of your life.

- You need to have a "why" that is going to be your motivating factor. What are you doing this for? There is no right or wrong answer when you are trying to change your mindset. Your why is your motivation, and it is the thing that keeps you going when you feel like giving up, or when you are struggling to stick to your plan. Your why can be the bikini you want to fit into, or it could be your cardiovascular health and cholesterol levels that you are hoping to improve. One of the best motivating factors that I found was my children. I realized that they are my *why*. I wanted to be around for a long time so that I could watch them grow, be a part of their lives, and watch them raise their own families. The stronger your *why*, the greater your determination and motivation will be to stay on track with your weight loss and health program. You also need to make sure that your motivation is in line with your goals. You can't be motivated by a contest that tests your strength when all you want to do is lose 10 lbs. The two need to coincide with each other and losing weight for health reasons is not the same as wanting to be the world's strongest woman.

- Set realistic goals for yourself. You need to know what you are hoping to achieve, and the most important part of this is making sure that your goal is realistic. You can't say that you hope to lose 20 lbs. in a week. That is neither realistic, attainable, nor healthy. You also cannot say that you hope to look like a bodybuilder in two weeks when you are only at the point of starting your workout and you are only able to lift a 5 lbs. dumbbell. If you are having trouble figuring out your goals, I have found that starting with how I feel is most important, and setting small goals is better than setting one giant goal that would otherwise leave me feeling disappointed.

- Focus on health education. As much as your body is unique, there are some universal health rules, like a salad and protein being healthier than takeout, that remain consistent and that will usually serve you well to know and keep in mind. Consult with health professionals if you find yourself at a point in the unknown where you don't know where the next step is. You need to have the proper education about your goals before you can move forward with your goals.

- Never underestimate the value of visualizations. Have you ever wondered why people create vision boards? They do this so that they can see exactly what they are hoping to achieve, and they can consciously and subconsciously begin setting plans in motion to achieve their goals. This is actually why creating a vision board is more effective than just setting a new year's resolution. If it is in front of you, it is not written on the first page of your diary or planner and is forgotten about. Instead, you see it and you are constantly reminded about how close or how much more you have to work to achieve it. The same goes for your physical body. Visualize yourself as a thinner and healthier version of yourself. The more you visualize it and picture it, the closer you will get to achieving this goal.

- Reward yourself... within reason. Life is meant to be enjoyed, and it can be enjoyed through small rewards. Think about how we get the weekend at the end of every week, or how we get an end-of-year vacation after working tirelessly the whole year. This is a great way of keeping ourselves motivated. But your year-end vacation doesn't usually turn into a five-month world tour. You do eventually have to head back to work and head back to reality before you start planning your next trip. Just in the same way that you will be sticking to a healthy eating plan and exercise regimen, give yourself a reward, especially when you see progress on the scale or with the tape measure. This means that you can have a cheat meal once a week, but it has to be within reason. If you lost five pounds, have a cheat meal to celebrate, but don't allow your cheat meal to be so great that it undoes everything you have done to achieve the five pounds loss.

- Create an action plan and have great support. It is easier to stay healthy when everyone in your home is actively working toward achieving the same lifestyle that you are working toward. It is also easy to follow a plan when you have something concrete in place. Follow exactly what you are going to eat each day, write it down, and tick it off as an accomplishment as you achieve it each day. Did you work out today? Tick it off your list. Did you stick to your eating plan all day? Tick it off your list. The sturdier your action plan, the less chance there is of you deviating from your plan.

- Get rid of your old habits. I am not saying to eat all the candy and unhealthy snacks in your home in one go so that you can start your healthy lifestyle. That is quite counter-productive. Instead, remove the unhealthy snacks from your shopping list and replace them with healthier alternatives. You will eventually begin establishing healthier habits and replacing the negative with the positive.

Each point helps you to cultivate a healthier mindset and when you have a healthy mind, you can have a healthy body. When you hear that people fought illnesses really well, they are not physically going to war and fighting their illnesses. They are fighting it with their mind, they are strengthening their mind and their immune systems, and their body follows along, becoming stronger and stronger. Your mind is a tool that leads the pack. Once you get that right, your path to healthy living and weight loss is pretty much established.

The Impact of Psychological Influences on the Body Weight Ratio

We've all been there—we have all had days where we come home from work and the day has been anything but easy. You've had curve balls thrown at you, confrontations to face, and a seemingly endless drive home. It all seemed to culminate with you in tears in the car on the way home. When you do eventually get home, it is dark, and you feel like you have forgotten what your house looks like in the daytime because you rarely ever spend any time at home. You kick off your shoes, pour yourself a glass of wine that is larger than life, take out the largest bag of chips that you can find in your pantry; you take out two candy bars because let's be honest, you deserve it, and you lay on the couch binge-watching your favorite show. The next thing you know, you are woken up by the silence because Netflix is still waiting for your response to its burning question of if you are still watching, and you are taken aback by the chocolate wrappers and empty bottle of wine that was just meant to be one glass. You sluggishly make your way to the bed, feeling just as bad as you did when you got home, but now it is because of guilt and shame rather than the horrible day you have had.

Now, this day could end here, the next morning you could wake up with an entirely different outlook and actually be ready to conquer the day. Or you could sink deeper and deeper, spiraling downwards into depression as each new day brings with it new challenges, which call for more comfort, that makes you feel worse, and that ultimately keeps you trapped in this cycle of sadness and depression. One can only wonder what effects this constant negative state of mind must have on one's body.

While psychology is a major component to be considered in weight gain, a bilateral effect happens where weight gain, in turn, affects an individual's psychology (Sutin, 2022). Studies have found that stress awareness and depression in women are significantly associated with weight gain (Jang et al., 2020).

People who are more likely to experience stress, or who are even more heightened and prone to stress on a daily basis are more likely to take in greater quantities of food, and the same has been reported on the relationship between depression and food intake, which ultimately leads to weight gain (Jang et al., 2020).

When you step away from weight gain alone and you look at people who are already obese, this impacts multiple psychological factors that lead to maintained obesity. People who are obese tend to face psychological effects of avoidance of their emotions, they have a low self-worth and body image, they tend to criticize themselves more often, they have negative core beliefs, and they often find themselves binge eating (Weight Matters, n.d.).

It is clear to see how intricately woven the mind and body actually are. If we can see the detrimental physical effects in terms of weight gain and obesity when women experience stress and depression, the inverse is clear to see. If you have a sound body and a sound mind, the chances of you being able to maintain your physical health are a lot higher.

But how do you keep yourself in a beneficial psychological capacity, especially when we live in a world that easily makes us prone to stress and depression, and that makes it easy to succumb to stress and depression? It is not as easy as telling yourself, "Stop stressing about work," or, "Don't be sad." If it were that easy, no one would be stressed or depressed.

There are certain things that you can do to treat stress and depression individually. When used effectively, it can be extended to target weight loss, and used with other methods to overcome the difficulty you may face with your weight. After all, weight affects your mental state and vice versa.

Stress

If you look at stress on its own, it is known that it is our body's response to external stimuli, and that is actually meant to keep us alive and out of danger. Stress becomes a problem when we begin focusing on things that are out of our control. For example, we need stress to meet a particular work deadline. And so, we work late at night, we put in extra hours, and we work a little harder to make sure that the outcome is not only great but that it is done on time. But then stress tends to take over and you find yourself stressing about irrational things. Eventually, you are in a state of frenzied stress because on your way to work, there was an accident, which caused you to face an unexpected delay, which led to you falling behind on your project with a looming deadline, which ultimately leads you to be convinced that you will lose your job. And just like that, your stress response goes into overdrive, thinking ten steps ahead when no one else around you is actually thinking that way.

The reason why stress makes it difficult to lose weight and maintain lost weight is because of one of two reasons. The first is that we develop unhealthy coping mechanisms, such as eating junk food, forgetting to drink water, and trying to fuel our bodies with things that are quick and convenient rather than healthy. We're also often so busy that we skip meals, get over-hungry, and stop at the nearest fast-food establishment for a quick and greasy burger. This is our behavior that is affecting our lack of weight loss, but it stems from stress.

The second reason is on a physiological level. When you are stressed, your body releases adrenaline and cortisol, which are hormones. Because of the hormones actively being released into our bodies, glucose, which is where your energy stems from, makes its way into your bloodstream. This is done to give you the energy you need to either fight-or-flight, which is the response activated by stress (Scott, 2019).

Now, it is in these moments that you will find yourself facing sugar cravings in the form of chocolates or chips because this is what gives you a quick energy kick that your body is actively craving. Because of this high sugar intake and the fact that you probably aren't running a marathon to burn off the sugar, your body ends up storing the sugar as fat. And to add a cherry on top, cortisol also lowers your metabolic rate, meaning that you burn fewer calories overall when stressed. So how do you overcome stress? There are a few exercises that you can start doing which, when used effectively, will allow you to control your stress, rather than your stress control you. First, when you find yourself in a moment of stress, stop for a second, and focus on your breathing. Take three to five deep breaths, allow them to fill your lungs, and you will find yourself feeling better and more in control. Breathing is a great grounding mechanism because it is something that happens so naturally and so continuously, but because it is an ever-present process in our life, focusing on it brings us back to the moment at hand, which stops us from thinking about something that hasn't happened yet, and that may not even happen.

You can also try to add some stretching and meditation into your routine as these practices, including active exercise, have been proven to lower stress levels. Be mindful of your acts, what you do in a day, and how you do it. If you are focused on what you are doing now, you tend to worry less about a future that you have no control over. If you are mindful of your everyday actions, you also tend to be more mindful of what you are eating and what you are putting into your body. When you are mindful of what you are putting into your body, you may find yourself taking in less alcohol, smoking less if you are a smoker, and avoiding medication in an attempt to indirectly calm yourself, all of which contribute to higher stress levels and are unhealthy coping mechanisms.

In relation to eating, there are some effective tools that can relate stress relief to eating. You see, when you consider that you cannot remove stress from your life, one thing you can do is control how you deal with and manage that stress. As you take on breathing, meditation, or stretching as a means to relieve stress, consider using exercise, even short bursts of ten jumping jacks and ten squats to get your blood flowing, as a way of actively reducing your stress. By doing exercise and getting some movement in, you actively release endorphins into your body and make yourself feel good. If you do have a hankering and cravings for some comfort food, there are healthier alternatives that you can choose, such as chips that are baked and not fried, or health bars instead of candy bars.

There is something that I was told often, and it worked wonders when I actually listened—our bodies mistake thirst for hunger, and for that reason, it is important to start every meal with a glass of cold water to make sure that you are not eating when you are actually hungry.

As mentioned, being mindful of what you eat, and even keeping track of what you eat in a food journal may actually put into perspective just how much you eat in a day.

Depression

The link between depression and weight gain and weight loss is extremely evident. There is no doubt that the link exists because the limbic system, which is the part of the brain that controls emotions, also controls the appetite (Bowers, 2012). While it is difficult to pinpoint whether depression leads to weight gain or weight loss, or whether weight gain and weight loss lead to depression, one thing that is certain is that the link is insurmountable.

Depression is tricky because it often goes hand-in-hand with weight loss and weight gain. While people who are depressed may not lose weight to a point where they are severely malnourished, there is a great chance of them gaining weight and becoming obese. On the flip side, however, people who suffer from an eating disorder, such as anorexia nervosa, bulimia nervosa, and binge eating disorder, often suffer from depression, and in the same way, people who are overweight or overly obese may approach their self-image with extreme negativity and get depressed because they don't like the way they look (Bowers, 2012).

With depression being as sensitive as it is yet extremely prominent, the general treatment usually follows the route of medication and therapy. However, there are people who prefer not to take medication to treat their depression, for fear that it may cause dependency or an altered personality state. But there are ways to combat depression naturally.

The first thing you can do is make an extra effort to stand up and walk around. This is really hard to do because when you are feeling depressed you want to stay in your comfort zone. But getting yourself moving can be profound and even representative of pulling yourself out from a rut that you may be stuck in. You are also going to find a way of meeting yourself where you are instead of setting up expectations for yourself that you know you can't meet.

Feeling depressed is a lot more than feeling blue or feeling sad. It can be all-consuming, which is why it is important that you actively do things and plan things for yourself that you know will bring you joy and comfort. Be careful, when you are facing depression, it is easy to think that sitting alone in the dark at home surrounded by unhealthy comfort food is doing something that makes you happy. It is not and although it is the comfort zone that you have created for yourself; it is not getting you into a healthy space.

When it comes to depression and weight management, you can't just treat one and hope that it remedies the other. Instead, you need to actively work toward remedying both aspects together and healing holistically. The starting point here is figuring out where depression and food intersect for you. You may find that when you are alone, or after interacting with a lot of people and your social battery is depleted, you tend to binge eat more. Finding the link between the two will help you target the problem at the root.

When you are actively moving, you will find yourself feeling better, and you will notice the physical changes that come with physical activity. And lastly, give yourself a break when you need it the most. Sometimes we take on too much and we find that diets, exercising, or just taking care of ourselves can't fit into our schedules. Your health should be a priority, not an option.

Permanent Weight Loss

The link between your state of mind and weight loss is evident and clear to see. Attention needs to be given to your mind for your body to have the right attention. You see, venturing down the path of weight loss is difficult. It takes constant hard work and constant effort, and it doesn't stop once your goal weight has been achieved. That is when you start working toward maintaining your weight and making sure that you don't fall back into old habits and pick up the weight again.

Once you get into the frame of mind that weight loss is not the once-off deal that fad diets promise, but rather actively working to maintain a goal and maintain your health, that's when the game changes. Get into the mindset of forever instead of for now.

Part of losing weight and keeping the weight off is being mindful of what stimuli you feed into your mind. There are things that you need to avoid and clear your mind of to align your focus on yourself and not on some unrealistic version of yourself. The first thing you need to do is be weary of what the internet is feeding into your mind. Getting thin quickly is not something that exists and if it does work, chances are that it comes with a hefty price to pay—which is usually in the form of your well-being.

You also need to be wary of social media and the impact it has on your mental and physical state. Many influencers may be out there trying to sell a version of yourself to you that will never exist. They are trying to sell you products that will help you look like them when, in reality, they are also focused on a healthy lifestyle instead of the empty promises that pills and supplements offer you. All that happens when you do try these influencer-endorsed products is that you don't achieve the body they have, for one of a thousand reasons, and that further affects your mental health, pushing you deeper and deeper into sadness and depression.

But all is not lost and if you find yourself inclined to try a weight loss product in the hopes that it helps you achieve and maintain your health goals, it is always best to first consult with a physician.

Remember, your mind matters, and your body can't get anywhere without its help.

Chapter 3:

The Impact of Physical Activity on

Your Weight Loss Journey

As I have been on my own journey and as I have helped others on their weight loss journey, I have come to learn that physical activity is either something you love or you hate, there is no in between. But whether you love it or hate it, it is an extremely important part of weight loss and weight management.

Everyone says that the perfect body is made in the kitchen, and while that is so true, the value of physical fitness greatly contributes to the effectiveness of your weight loss. For example, there was a time when I was on a diet that promised quick results with zero exercise. I was told that within two weeks I was going to have my dream body. In retrospect, these were all red flags. Nevertheless, I went for it, and I stuck to this diet really well. I was really committed and diligent, and it proved to be true. By the end of the first week, I had dropped the bulk of my weight. But by the middle of the second week, I noticed that the weight loss had stopped. There was no plan or guidance for what should happen after the two weeks were up and by the time the diet came to an inevitable end, I had picked up all the weight I had just lost, with a few extra pounds for good measure.

With that being said, I have also been on the opposite end of the spectrum where I worked out insanely hard every day for months on end and I saw absolutely no difference because I chose to eat the worst foods around. I ate everything that was unhealthy with the excuse that it is alright, I will burn it off at the gym. This did not happen, and all my attempts at the gym were futile.

The reality is that physical exercise, which is made up of a combination of strength, cardio, and endurance training, is integral to the overall health and success of your weight loss journey, but most importantly, it is important in maintaining your desired weight. Dieting and reducing your food intake without engaging in physical activity is entirely useless and futile, and sometimes, even changing your eating habits is not the solution at all.

If, with a new eating plan, you find that you have lost weight but the weight loss plateaus, which is expected to happen, the only way to kickstart your progress once again is to maintain your eating habits and add in physical activity. This allows your body to get to a point where you are able to change your body and lose weight, but also maintain it in the long run. Losing weight without any physical activity is not sustainable, and this is exactly why it seems so easy to gain weight, but it seems so difficult to lose weight.

Yes, what you eat is important, but just as important is what you do with your body physically.

Physical Activity For Beginners

I have found many of the women that I have coached and worked with tell me that they refuse to do strength training because they don't want to be built like a man with giant muscles, and this was a misconception that needed to be shattered. Muscle helps your body burn fat, and because you are the one that sets your goal and works toward achieving your goal if you do not want to have giant biceps, there are ways for you to achieve and maintain the perfect muscle mass needed in your body without looking like you could enter a bodybuilder competition.

On the other hand, I have had other people tell me that they refuse to do cardio because they hate being that much out of breath with the pain forming in their chest after intense and vigorous training.

Now, the thing is, you can't do only one aspect of training and expect to see holistic results, just in the same way that you can't only change your diet or only exercise—the two are interlinked and interdependent. The reality is that physical activity can be really hard, and because it is hard, it can be easy to lose motivation. But that is why I encourage people, including myself, to find and do exercises that I actually enjoy doing. Because although they are going to make my muscles ache, I have such a great time doing them that I don't even mind the ache that comes with it.

As a beginner or someone who hasn't engaged in much physical activity before, it is important not to throw yourself into the deep end. Not only will you quickly grow to despise exercise, but you will also find yourself getting injured quickly, which will ultimately lead to further setbacks.

Exercise is not about heading into a gym and doing whatever you see the person in front of you doing. It requires you to work from the bottom up and do exercises in a way that doesn't cause more harm than good. Getting an injury during exercise is common when you take on more strain than you can handle. Your body literally buckles under the pressure, and just when you were starting your exercise routine, you now need to stop for your body to heal. This can sometimes set you back for weeks.

Moving from a sedentary lifestyle where you engage in no physical activity at all is a great starting point because you can only move upwards from there. Making sure you get regular movement at this point is far better than making sure you do any form of intense strength training. If you find yourself sitting for most of the day, stand up at least every hour, even if you are setting an alarm to remind you, and walk around your desk and space for two minutes.

There was a time when I noticed and watched not only my own behaviors but that of others who also complained that they don't have time for physical activity. Yes, they would be constantly busy, but when they were hungry or needed a snack, they would take out a bag of chips and a candy bar, turn on a five-minute-long YouTube video, and engage in an unhealthy break as opposed to a healthy alternative. The healthy alternative that was actively put to the test was to replace the unhealthy snack with apple slices (two apples if they were particularly hungry) and walk around the office space or their desk for two minutes. The exact same five-minute break was spent in entirely different ways. Guess who had more energy when they had to get back to work five minutes later?

Small, regular movements are a great way for starting out, and eventually, with consistency, you will hunger for more... not snacks, but physical movements. The reason why I mention work explicitly is that when you really think about it, home and work are the two places that occupy the most time and space in our lives. If you can find a way of incorporating physical activity into this part of your day, you are bound to achieve small successes. Move around your workspace and your home space, and if you are one of the lucky few people who get to work from home, you may find yourself having a little more freedom to incorporate more physical activity into your days, like a walk around your garden or even your neighborhood.

Do you know what is a great form of physical activity that doesn't even feel like working out? If you have kids, playing with them outside, playing tag, running around, rolling on the grass, laughing, and tumbling are great ways of getting the physical exercise in, but also, even better, you get to truly bond and enjoy time with your little one, which really makes it one of the greatest forms of exercises.

The aim of slowly incorporating exercise into a sedentary lifestyle is to do it in a way that doesn't take away any time from the routine you have already established for yourself. The primary reason why people say they can't work out or exercise is that they are too busy, so if introducing physical activity is going to make them feel like their day is cut even shorter than it already is, it is going to be near impossible to stick to their workout. Instead, you want it to seamlessly meld into your established lifestyle so that you don't feel inconvenienced by your health.

There are small things that you can do to achieve this. Park a mile away from your office and walk the rest of the way to your office. By the end of each day, you would have walked a total of two miles to and from your office, just by changing where you park.

We all know the feeling of searching for a parking spot closest to the mall entrance so that we don't have to walk far. Next time, gracefully accept any parking you can get and if you have any shopping bags to take to your car, if it is within reason, ditch the shopping cart and work your arm muscles.

One way to actively achieve a slight increase in your physical activity is to try and do more footwork and less work on the chair. The way life is moving, and the way many people's jobs are structured requires you to spend exorbitant amounts of time at a desk. But as humans, we were not designed to sit for eight hours a day. It is important to take five trips to the copier to get in the movement you would otherwise forget to do. If it is possible for you to stand and work on occasion, do it… your body will thank you for it later.

Creating a Schedule to Form a Routine

Just in the same way that planning meals limits the amount of fast food and takeout you may consume, establishing a realistic schedule that includes and incorporates physical activity is one of the best ways of making sure you include and stick to physical activity in your day.

It is easy to fall into the excuse of not having enough time to do something in the day, but when you have earmarked and set time aside dedicated to a task, you are accountable to yourself and to the looming to-do list and schedule that is staring you in the face.

Ideally, you want to form healthy habits, but how do these habits form? Through mindful practices, which means being conscious and aware of what you are doing in the day instead of floating through life on auto-pilot, you can develop healthy habits which seamlessly fit into your daily routine.

Habits and routine go hand-in-hand, and one forms part of the other. You can't develop a healthy habit without making a mindful and conscious effort to include it in your day, and you can't build a routine without having a set place for your habitual practices.

So let us start looking at forming a habit. We know that it takes around 21 days to form a habit, but it takes a lot longer to actually stick to the habit. It takes a lot longer for the habit to become second nature. It is for that reason that creating a very specific goal for physical activity is important. Be realistic with your time before you set this goal. If you are someone who doesn't usually exercise, and doesn't particularly enjoy exercising, then saying you want to exercise every day is very vague and is more likely to lead to avoidance than actually sticking to it.

Instead, you are going to set a specific goal such as, "I am going to do exercise or some form of physical activity for 15 minutes in the morning before I start my workday." This is a specific goal in a defined time frame that makes it easier to stick to. You don't give yourself the opportunity of postponing physical activity for a later time that may never come. Instead, you have a specific time in which to complete your physical activity.

Ideally, you want your habit to be cue-based. Let's be honest, we are human, and we forget. It is easy for an entire day to go by without us thinking about our workout and sometimes, we do just forget. If you have a cue or something that triggers a reminder, you are more likely to remember what you are hoping to do, and the same goes for workouts. While you can tell yourself that after your morning coffee you will do your exercise, I am a fan of a good old-fashioned alarm that sounds consistently as a reminder every day. It removes the mental load of trying to remind myself to do things, but I still get the much-needed cue and reminder to exercise.

As previously mentioned, if you are going to stick to exercise and activity, you need to make it enjoyable. If you absolutely despise burpees, try to replace them with a more enjoyable activity because I guarantee you that it is going to be hard to form that habit, let alone stick to it.

Yes, we want structure, we want cue-based plans, and we want specific times for specific tasks. But let's be honest, there are days where we are sick, or our kids are sick, or we have to catch an early flight, or we have family over, and this stops us from sticking to our routine and stands in the way of forming our habit. Yes, we want it to become second nature and a natural, automatic part of our day, but feeling stuck and tied down by a task can easily make you feel tied down and obliged to do something you are meant to want to do. When you are in the early stages of forming and creating your habit, switch times around every now and then. See what it feels like for your body to exercise in the evening rather than in the morning so if you face a roadblock in your routine, you do have an alternate option.

And lastly, I only realized the importance and the major difference that support makes when I worked out alone at home, and when I signed up for a spin class with 20 other like-minded individuals. The support and community feeling that you get from others is enough in itself to keep you motivated, not to mention that you become accountable to many other people, instead of just to yourself, your schedule, and your alarms.

Now that you have built a habit, and you have established a daily schedule (including weekends because many people tend to forget about schedules and routines on weekends), you can seamlessly integrate physical activity into your daily routine. It is important to know that a daily routine on Monday may look different from your routine on Tuesday, but the fact that you have the opportunity to establish a routine that suits you each day makes it more likely for you to stick to your routine no matter how different each day looks from each other.

Exercise as part of a regular and habitual routine increases the number of calories that you burn in a day, and guess what? That greatly contributes to weight loss (CDC, 2020). Yes, your body will get used to the exercise you are doing, and it may "plateau," but when this happens, you can increase the intensity or duration, or you can continue doing what you are doing to maintain the weight you are currently at.

Additionally, other habits that you can incorporate into your daily, weekly, and monthly lifestyle that can help you lose weight are (Holmes Place, 2018):

- Plan everything, your meals, your routine, everything. When you have a plan in place, there's a lower chance of you deviating from the path that will lead you to your goal.

- Don't shop hungry. Whether you stop for supplies weekly or monthly, you are more likely to add that bag of chips or that extra candy bar into your cart if you are hungry than if you are shopping on a full tummy and sticking to the list that you planned.

- Be mindful about what you put into your mouth and make sure not to skip meals, especially not breakfast.

- Don't swap out one candy bar with a different flavor that you also like; instead, make healthy swaps. Try a healthy trail mix or nuts instead of candy.

- Try a smaller dinner plate, but this also means downsizing your portion size to accommodate your dinner plate instead of creating a mountain of food on a very tiny plate.

- And lastly, walk anywhere and everywhere that's possible. Walking is the best form of exercise, so try to include it in your day in any way possible and as much as possible.

While you are busy scheduling and planning your daily routine, make sure to schedule a workout and plan your meals for the day, make sure to include a plan for rest days and cheat days. Rest days are important for long-term workouts, which is exactly what we are going for. You can have one or two rest days a week, depending on your goals and how much your body is able to handle. It is important to stay attuned to what you are feeling and if you are feeling overly strained, it may be your body telling you it needs a rest. Schedule your rest days, but I personally try to avoid scheduling my rest days and cheat days on the same day. If I am having a cheat day, I try to work out on that day, so I don't feel unnecessarily guilty.

When you are establishing a plan for yourself, remember that it is for yourself. It doesn't have to fit anyone else's idea of perfection as long as it works for you and it is something you can commit to in the long run. Ultimately, without physical activity, weight loss can never be sustained. It doesn't have to be an unrealistic amount of time dedicated to strenuous exercise. You would be surprised what five or ten minutes of exercise can do for you each day. You would be even more surprised about how good you feel after the positive hormones are surging through your veins.

Chapter 4:

Overcoming Hidden Barriers to

Achieve Your Fitness and Health

Goals

Many people encounter many barriers on their weight loss and health journey. Sometimes, it is them trying to figure out their body type, sometimes it is juggling chronic illnesses like diabetes that impact their weight loss, and other times, it is a lack of knowledge and understanding of the components that contribute to weight loss that serves as an invisible barrier.

Let's be honest, with all the "must do's" and "have to do's" that diets and weight loss programs come with, it is difficult to keep track of what you need to put into your body. With all the recommendations of what you need to put into your body on a daily basis, even to lose weight, it might seem like a lot to take in. Not only is it difficult to understand why you need to consume so much food but understanding each food group can be overwhelming. But it is important to know what the diet and food-related terminology are so that you can know and understand why you need to put these things into your body.

You've probably heard words like carbs, proteins, and fats thrown around, and if you have heard these words, you have probably also heard that carbs are the sinful foods that you need to entirely rid from your diet and that you basically only need to consume proteins. But this can ultimately cause more harm than good to your weight loss journey.

Before you head blindly into cutting out carbs and other food groups because you have heard that it makes you gain weight, you should probably learn what each of these food groups bring to your health and diet, and you should probably know what they mean. Having the knowledge will assist you in making the best decisions for your eating plan and getting the most out of the foods you eat.

You will see many health tips recommending that you eat freshly prepared meals because you know exactly what is going into them and that you try to incorporate as many food groups into your daily food intake as possible. These tips will also include advice telling you not to skip breakfast and that breakfasts and other meals are made up of wholesome foods.

So let us understand some of the terminologies that are important for your health and weight loss journey. In attempting to eat a balanced meal for weight loss, you do need to be mindful of what you are putting in your body. Your meals, therefore, need to be balanced so that you are providing your body with all the nutrients it needs for survival and to function optimally. There are five food groups that you need to include in your eating plan and meal plan to lose weight.

- The first food group that you need for weight loss is carbohydrates. Yes, the very thing you may have been avoiding is the same thing that you need to lose weight. While other food groups feed your body and get absorbed by your body, carbs are actually your primary source of energy. Ultimately, carbs should make up half of your daily calorie intake because this is what your body will burn as energy. However, there are good carbs and bad carbs. You see, when people tell you to avoid carbs, they usually mean to avoid the heavily processed carbs that come in the form of fried potato chips or tortilla flatbreads that are slathered in thick heaps of garlic butter. There are also carbs that contain excessive amounts of sugar such as bread and white rice (Decathlon Blog, 2022). You need to be mindful of the types of carbs you are consuming.

- The next food group that you need to consume for weight loss is protein. I am sure you have heard of this one before on your weight loss journey, and I am sure you know why protein is so needed in your body. If you don't know why then allow me to explain. While carbs are the fuel your body uses during daily activity, protein is the actual food for your body. Your muscles require protein, and the greater your muscle mass, the faster you will metabolize fat. Protein helps in repairing your cells and your muscles help in producing new cells and is paramount for the healthy development of your bones, skin, and many other organs. When you take in the right amount of protein, your body will absorb it rather than expend it. This means that your muscle mass and strength will increase, you will notice a reduction in your appetite, you will burn more calories, and you won't find yourself craving as many candy bars as you once used to. Because protein feeds your body and your muscles, it doesn't crave extra food because your body is technically full. The quick-fix meals you are so desperately craving are no longer needed because your protein intake is enough to keep your body full.

- The next important food group that is extremely important for weight loss is fiber. Now, you may roll your eyes at me, or you may be reading this with dread in your heart thinking of all the fiber cereals that are currently lining your kitchen shelves but that you just can't bring yourself to eat. Reading this may feel like utter misery because you think you have to subject yourself to these bland breakfasts. But that's not true. At the foundation of understanding why fiber is so important in your diet means first knowing what it does for you. Our gut can either be healthy or unhealthy. Now, you may have heard people say that they can eat anything, milk doesn't upset their stomach, but they do face constipation. Well, constipation, diarrhea, bloating, gas, and heartburn, are all signs of an unhealthy gut. But what makes your gut unhealthy? Your gut has an internal microbiome that consists of good and helpful bacteria, and bad bacteria. These bacteria need to be balanced for you to have a healthy gut. The second they are unbalanced favoring the bad bacteria, or if the levels of both good and bad bacteria in your gut drop too low, your gut is unhealthy and can lead to the abovementioned symptoms. When your gut is healthy and it is favoring the good bacteria, you may find yourself having healthy and regular bowel movements, more energy, mental clarity, and good reactions to food. You may also notice that milk won't make you bloated and that stress won't really affect your tummy. But what does fiber have to do with your gut health? Well, fiber serves as nourishment for your gut bacteria which allows your gut lining to stay intact. This maintains the integrity of your stomach lining, preventing your stomach's bacteria from turning your stomach lining into food. It also improves your digestion and reduces constipation. Now, back to the bran flakes cereal that makes you cringe just thinking about it—this does not need to be your only source or a source of fiber for you at all. Instead, you can up your intake of green leafy vegetables, fruits like apples and pears, oats, and more which are great sources of fiber and can even help manage your blood sugar and cholesterol levels (Decathlon Blog, 2022).

- The next food group that you need for your weight loss journey, and it is probably going to shock you, is fat. For the longest time, I thought fat was the greasy white stuff left in the pan after I had cooked bacon. But that is not the only kind of fat that exists. Yes, the type of fat or grease left behind after cooking bacon is not the healthy kind and is usually the type of fat that causes high cholesterol. But not all fats are bad fats. In fact, fats should make up around 20% of your diet plan (Decathlon Blog, 2022). This doesn't mean that you should eat butter straight from the tub, but instead, you can find fats such as omega-3 fatty acids from fish, and you can find polyunsaturated and monounsaturated fats from dark chocolate, eggs, avocado, nuts, and a variety of unsweetened nut butters (Leonard, 2018).

- Lastly, you need vitamins and minerals which make up an important part of an eating plan for weight loss. Vitamins and minerals are not just supplements you take to stop yourself from getting sick and that you use to keep your bones and teeth healthy. Instead, they play an important part in making sure your muscular function stays up to par, and they assist in keeping your metabolism running smoothly. And while there are an endless amount of off-the-shelf supplements that can provide you with all the vitamins and minerals that you need, getting them from food sources is getting them in a way that your body knows best how to absorb.

On your journey to weight loss, you may also find yourself constantly reminded to drink water. Staying hydrated is such an important part of weight loss and overall health, but sometimes it is easily forgotten. I can tell you how many times I have had a busy day full of running errands and before I know it, it is 3 p.m. and I haven't had more than a few sips of water. Not to mention that there was a part of me that used to actively avoid drinking water when I had a busy day ahead because I knew how often I was going to need to run to the bathroom.

When I started my own journey, I also found myself actively trying to avoid or minimize my water intake for what retrospectively seems like a very strange reason. Early on in my weight loss journey, before I had the plethora of information that I have now, I found myself leaning heavily on what the scale said. Firstly, the scale is not the best measurement of weight loss, and secondly, I found my weight fluctuating by almost three pounds on a daily basis. I learned that the more water I drank, the heavier I appeared on the scale, and because the scale mattered so much to me, I found myself drinking less and less water. This was an issue that I carried with me for a long time until I got my mindset right and stopped attaching such a great value to the scale in my life. It was then that I truly began feeling the beneficial effects of water in my life, and I realized just how great it was to feel hydrated.

The Biggest Myths About Muscle Building and Body Toning

As you become better acquainted with the world of health and fitness and as you start learning more about your body and doing things that will ultimately better your health, you will learn for yourself just how false some of the information you were previously fed actually was. The reality is that there is an endless amount of information out there, and it is not to say that someone is false about advertising quick weight loss strategies that happen quickly without much effort. But the reality is that eating soup for 14 days may have worked for them, but it may not work for you. They may have lost up to 10 lbs. in those 14 days, but they may fail to mention the side effects that they experienced after or during those 14 days. So, while there are endless "quick fixes" and fast weight loss methods, there is also the way that takes time and effort but that works across the board for anyone that may try it.

As you go down your own unique path, you may find it easier for you to decipher what is real and what myths exist in weight loss and building up fitness. But to make that somewhat easier for you, allow me to share what I have learned on my journey as well.

The True Meaning of Body Toning and Shaping

You may have heard many people say that they want to tone up and get in shape so that they can be skinnier for the summer. But the reality is that each of these components that they are talking about (toning, shaping, and being skinny) are very different.

Let's first look at body toning. Toning refers to the muscle's ability to contract and release in terms of reflexes and ability. Muscle tone is something that can be gained and lost. For example, if someone is very ill and they are bedridden, temporarily or even permanently, they will have reduced muscle tone and it may make things like walking a lot harder. However, you can increase your muscle tone by working out and shaping them. Obviously, the bigger and more defined you want them to be, you will work harder to shape specific focus areas. It has become a point of humor where many people say that you shouldn't miss leg day. People's legs may not seem to be in shape because they probably don't give them the attention they deserve.

While shaping does happen depending on how much you concentrate on working on a specific muscle group, there are other cosmetic ways of shaping one's body such as by using implants, Botox injections, and skin tightening methods.

What Does Body Sculpting Mean?

We all want to look like a Greek goddess with a body that is worthy to have prose and poetry written about its pure perfection. But the reality is that sometimes our 5' 2", wide stature doesn't allow us to have legs for days and our wide hips make it almost impossible to see the well-defined abs we may have been working on for months. It is easy to get dismayed by this and it is to be deterred from the ultimate goal you may have had in mind. No, you won't have the physique of a model, but you will have the physique of a healthier you. For some people, this is not enough, and many people find themselves seeking medical assistance to get the body they desire. And that is what body contouring is. It is a process whereby medical or surgical procedures are used to reshape a specific part of the body. As mentioned above, it may involve skin tightening or implants, but it may also involve liposuction or the redistribution of fat in a specific part of the body to make other parts appear fuller than others or to minimize the appearance of cellulite. It can even be the removal of excess skin, which many people feel the need to do after dramatic weight loss.

While this may appear to be a quick fix and a viable option for anyone who can afford it, the effects may not be long-lasting, and the healing process can take an extremely long time. Also, any form of surgery or medical procedure comes with a risk, and this risk may be mitigated or even non-existent if you consider weight loss in the natural sense of the word.

Lifting Weights Will Make You Bulky

While I have touched on this previously, it is a great misconception that many people have about strength and weight training making them bulky. Many people think that the only way to lose weight is to focus on cardio and ignore the weights until it is time to tone up. I was also a victim of this false notion, and I was of the firm belief that I had to lose all my weight first, watching it melt away like butter before I worked on muscle definition. What I only found out much later is that you need to build muscle because building muscle loses weight.

It is very difficult to become "bulky" by accident. When you think of pro athletes who compete in weightlifting or bodybuilding competitions, their journeys aren't by accident or overnight. Instead, it takes excessive hard work, determination, and extreme focus to get to that point. Picking up a 5 lb. or even a 10 lb. dumbbell is not going to get you to an overly bulky stage. Unless that is your aim and your goal, you can safely lift weights to lose weight without qualifying for a heavyweight bodybuilding competition.

The More You Exercise, the Better

This myth is actually a scary one that can do more harm than good. You know how they say that too much of a good thing can be bad? I think they were talking about over-exercising. Look, we know the benefits of working out and exercising, it has been covered in length in this book already and you have probably seen the benefits of exercise outside of this book for however long you have been working on your health or trying to lose weight. But what rarely gets pointed out or discussed is the detrimental effects of over-exercising or working out too much.

Yes, there is such a thing as too much exercise and while it does release endorphins and all those feel-good hormones, it can actually cause a hormone imbalance because you are not giving your hormones and your body a chance to get back to baseline and re-regulate. Over and above the hormonal damage that it can inflict on your body, you may find yourself not being able to perform at the same level you used to. This is because your body is just tired and needs a break. When you overexert yourself, you have a greater chance of getting injured. You work your muscles too hard; you don't give them a chance to recover and you essentially have a kink in your armor that is prone to injury. And then, when you do get injured, because you don't allow your body a chance to rest, your recovery time becomes longer and longer, and now you are kept away from the one thing you gave so much attention to—working out.

But these are just the physical and physiological effects of over-exercising. You may also face negative mental effects such as being constantly tired, feeling like all you want to do is rest, not having as much energy, being depressed, having mood swings, and even facing difficulties sleeping.

You Need to Workout for the Muscle Burn

Feeling the muscle burn is great, it not only makes you feel like you are doing something right, but you realize that you have muscles albeit hidden beneath some extra layers. But that is not all that working out is about, and sometimes that isn't even what you need.

In most cases, people who are extremely overweight will do a healthy combination of cardio and weight training. The weight training that they are doing is not just yet targeted to any specific muscle group but is rather used as a way to slightly build muscle so that their muscle and cardio workouts can work in tandem to lose weight. It is only at a later stage when it is needed and necessary, they will focus on exercising specific muscle groups and it is then that they can chase the burn.

Doing the Wrong Exercise is Worse Than no Exercise At All

This is the one myth that is kind of worthy of a laugh. Believing this myth is having the same concept of wanting to lose weight and eat healthier so instead of fighting the craving for one candy bar, you eat all five candy bars that are in your pantry. If you consider that the alternative to the "wrong" exercise is no exercise at all, which seems like the better option?

Let us start at the beginning and look at the concept of a wrong exercise. Yes, there are wrong ways to do an exercise, but I personally don't think that there are wrong exercises. Anything that gets your heart rate up and gets your blood pumping is intrinsically good for you and beneficial to you. It can seem like exercises are wrong when they appear to be ineffective, but in such cases, I would recommend you go back to the drawing board and consider if your eating habits match the workout you are doing. Doing all cardio and no weight training isn't technically wrong, it is just not ideal. So, while you can't do the wrong exercises, you can optimize your workouts in a way that will allow for holistic weight loss and health gain.

Training Without Proper Guidance is Absolutely Useless

This myth follows the similar concept of no exercise being better than the "wrong" exercises. Yes, having the proper guidance and training can quickly optimize your workout, it can teach you the proper form of some workouts, and provides a greater sense of accountability because you have someone to be accountable to and who can help you on your journey. But when you consider that there are so many people out there who are getting guidance from social media and YouTube videos, it is easy to realize that wanting proper guidance can be used as an excuse to avoid exercising at all.

In most cases, you don't even need to get elaborate or overly fancy with your workouts and you would be surprised at how effective simple workouts that require no guidance can actually be.

A healthy combination of knowledge and activity is bound to set you on a path that allows you to have a better relationship with your body. Knowing what each food group is, how it benefits and contributes to your body, and quickly filtering out the lies from the truths when it comes to fitness is the best way of creating a holistic way of following a weight loss journey and heading down a path of health and happiness.

Chapter 5:

Setting Goals That Will Motivate

You On Your Journey

Goals, goals, goals. They are a very important part of success. After all, how will you work toward your dream or success if you don't know what that dream is? Goals are important for several reasons, the first of which is that it gives you the opportunity to try and test new behaviors to achieve this goal. For example, if you have never worked out a day in your life before and you decide that your goal is to lose five pounds, you are going to undertake a behavior that you have never before pursued—you are going to exercise and change your eating habits. This is something new that is triggered by the goal you have set in place. Your goal is what keeps you motivated when you find motivation a bit hard to come by. Trust me, those days will come, the days where you would rather sleep or watch TV, or eat that candy bar instead of working out, or the days where you would rather order takeout than cook a healthy meal. When those days come, your goals are sometimes the only thing that keeps you motivated.

When you consider that achieving something is entirely abstract and unique to you, having goals in place gives you a way of measuring your progress. I'm going to be brutally honest with you—as great as it is to have like-minded people supporting you and to whom you feel accountable, the reality is that everyone is on their own journey, and you are the only person that your goal matters to. Having a goal means you know where your starting point was and it gives you a way and means of measuring your progress by comparing your present self to your past self, with the idea of your future self (goal) in mind.

The best type of goals that you can set for yourself, in any area of your life, are SMART goals. SMART goals stand for:

- Specific

- Measurable

- Achievable

- Relevant

- Time-bound

If you thought setting your weight loss goals was going to be as easy as thinking *I want to be 20 lbs. lighter by Christmas*, then you are in for a surprise. When I work with clients, what I found to be most effective for myself was dedicating some time to set and establish the parameters of our goals. Setting a goal in your mind might be great for your daily to-do list and for what you are hoping to achieve by the end of the day, but for long-term goals, it is going to be hard to wrap your head around the specifics of your goal. So, when I draft a SMART goal plan, I grab a pen and a piece of paper and I get to it.

The great thing about SMART goals is the same methodology can be used for your personal relationships, holiday plans, professional goals, fitness goals, and even hobbies. It can even be used for your financial goals. But I am going to show you what's the best way to establish SMART goals for your weight loss journey (Boogaard, 2021).

- Specific—the key to achieving any goal is knowing exactly what it is you are hoping to achieve. When you are specific about your goal, you are going to answer three questions: 1) What needs to be accomplished? 2) Who is responsible for making sure this goal is accomplished? 3) What steps do you need to take to make this goal a reality? In terms of your weight loss, the answer to these questions would be first, you want to accomplish weight loss. We can always add muscle toning later on because goals are constantly adapting (after all, once you achieve your weight loss, you need something else to work toward). The second answer will be that you are responsible for accomplishing this goal. Unfortunately, you cannot hire someone you can delegate certain exercises to in order for you to lose weight. Lastly, you need to define the steps that you are going to take to lose weight. It is here where you will include not just that you are going to eat healthier and exercise, but you are going to state exactly what you are hoping to eat, preferably in the form of a meal plan and a detailed exercise regimen for each day.

- Measurable—attaching a measurement to your goal makes it easier for you to achieve because you can measure your progress, how far you have come, and how much more you have to go. You can define how many pounds you are hoping to lose overall, or how many pounds you are hoping to lose each week; you can define how many inches you are hoping to lose around your waist and other parts of your body, or you could even define how many dress sizes you are hoping to come down. Perhaps you have an outfit that you are hoping to fit into. You can use that as a measurement of your progress.

- Achievable—we know from the get-go that just like getting rich quick schemes, quick weight loss is neither sustainable, healthy, or in some cases realistic. This is why you need to set achievable goals. For example, let's say that you were hoping to lose 2 lbs. a week on the new weight loss regimen you are on. After two or three weeks you realize that you are only able to realistically lose 1 lb. a week. This is fine and it shouldn't deter you or make you feel like you are never going to achieve your goal. Instead, you should adjust your goal to accommodate what is achievable for you and your body. Remember that we are trying to be realistic. You don't want to lose 10 lbs. in a week. Setting unrealistic goals is just going to make you feel worse when you don't achieve them even though they weren't attainable in the first place.

- Relevant—in the short term and in the long term, you want your goal to be relevant. What this means is that you need to have a sound and study why behind the goal you are setting. We have already covered this in previous chapters but when your reasoning behind your goal is sound, it makes it easier to stick to it. Let's make a comparison of two motivating factors. Your motivating factor can be trying to get into a bikini for the summer or that you just found out you are borderline diabetic, and your cholesterol is quite high. These are two very good motivating factors to lose weight. However, if by the time summer comes, you have not met your goal, you may have realized that you look great in a one-piece swimsuit instead of the two-piece swimsuit and you may abandon your goal altogether. However, you consistently work toward a healthy lifestyle if your motivating factor is your long-term health. In such an example, the relevance of the first motivation was short-lived and quickly abandoned. The second motivation is relevant for a longer period of time and is more likely to keep you motivated.

- Time-bound—lastly, you want to make sure that you give yourself a deadline by when you would like to achieve your goal. Not having a timeline attached to your goal allows you to float almost without purpose in a futile attempt to achieve that goal. If you don't set a time for your weight loss, you may find yourself gaining more weight before you actually begin working toward losing weight because you are under the false impression that you have all the time in the world. Now, something that you may be wondering and that I also wondered and had a fear of was what if I don't meet my goal by the stipulated time? Well, goals are meant to be adjusted. If you find that you have fallen short of your goal or you have far surpassed your goal in a specific time, then you can take that into consideration when you set your next goals.

Understanding Your Ideal Body

To set your ideal goals, you need to get into the mind of your future self. You need to understand and visualize what your ideal body looks like. But remember that you are not putting your head on someone else's body. You are working with what you have and working toward getting the best out of it. You want to give yourself a specific target that is tailor-made for you and not just because someone else has achieved that specific goal.

You also want to make sure that you understand your body and your natural inclinations as a person before you set a goal for yourself. This will help you know what is realistic and achievable for you rather than just feeling your way around blindly. It will also make your goals more realistic rather than just allowing yourself to feel like you are failing.

You also need to be wise about the influences you let into life. There are people that are going to bring you down, people that are going to lift you up, and people that you may not want to be with because although they motivate you, the comparison makes you feel like a failure. There are also those people who are going to be fully aware of your goals, and they are still going to point out how slow or little progress you have made. Ideally, when you have a mindset on a goal, you need to be alert to the influences that are showing up in your life. You need to be your own greatest influence.

With these goals that you have established, and the detailed game plan that you have developed for yourself, in the back of your mind, something that should serve as a constant reminder is the fact that you are going to do whatever it takes to return to your ideal state of health. While short-lived may be the goal, it is important to remind yourself that your reason is to achieve an ideal state of health, and weight loss is ultimately a byproduct of healthy living.

The True Reason Behind Achieving Your Goals

We all have our major motivating factors. As I previously mentioned, for me, that motivation is my children, but along the way, I have had to take my wins and my losses even with them as my greatest motivating factor. What this means is that there is a possibility that I don't achieve my goal, that I fall off the wagon, or that I learn the hard way that my goals were not realistic. My kids are still going to be my motivation, but the dynamic somewhat changes. You see, setting a goal and having something to work toward is always going to be far more important than actually achieving my goal. Don't get me wrong, achieving a goal is a magnificent feeling, but if you don't achieve your goal, it can come with intense demotivation. That is why I have quite consistently been mentioning revisiting and adapting your goals. Part of your goal-setting plan is going to be a reassessment and reevaluation of your goals every three weeks. I have found this period of time to work quite perfectly not just for myself but for others too. The reason is that in three weeks, you can experience quite substantial results. And small results are still results. Every three weeks, while you are working toward achieving your goal, you are also going to be taking an intel of data such as how you feel, how much progress have you made thus far, and how you need to change and adapt your goal accordingly. Setting, resetting, and constantly adjusting your goal is going to keep you motivated, and working toward something without falling off track.

When you set out on your game plan and start putting your plan into action, you need to take and manage your goal in small, bite-sized pieces. This will allow you to achieve little milestones within your goal process, making you feel more accomplished rather than working toward something that seems so far out of reach. Approaching your goal in small portions makes it feel more achievable because you are ticking off accomplishments on the way.

You also need to be understanding of your body. If achieving your goal means breaking every part of your mind, body, and soul, then your goal seriously needs to be reevaluated. Along the road toward achieving your goal you also need to sift out the myths from the truths and most importantly, you need to realize that working hard toward achieving a goal can be fun, can bring you joy, and you don't need to be confined by the constraints that you have created for yourself. When you set your goals, know that you will have moments to celebrate, moments to take a break, and cheat days and remind yourself that these are all a part of the process of achieving your goals.

Chapter 6:

The First Physical Changes in Your

Weight Loss Journey

Everyone has a starting point. Whether you have been doing gymnastics since you could walk or whether you only began doing physical activity at 30, everyone has a fitness starting point. At some stage, even the greatest athletes were beginners and that is the comfort you can take in your starting point.

In this chapter, we are going to delve into the exercises you will be pursuing as a beginner, you will figure out how to know what works for you, what is healthy discomfort, and what is a sign that you should pause immediately, and most importantly, you will learn how to stick to what the exercises you have started.

Winning the Game From Within

As much as exercise is an outward physical activity, you need to get your head in the game, and you need to get your mindset right. Yes, we have spoken about getting your mindset in the right place for weight loss, but now, you need to get it into the place of putting your plan into physical activity and making the sacrifice of time to get to a place where you can do your daily physical activity.

The odds are going to forever be stacked in your favor, provided you use them correctly and you make the most out of what you are given.

For example, if you work a full-time job, you have a husband and kids to take care of, and a house that you are constantly working toward making a home, chances are you are going to need to create a time in your day dedicated to exercise. But we are mere humans, we cannot fabricate time out of anything. This is going to mean going to bed a little later or waking up a little earlier, so you don't lose out on what is most important to you, and that you find space for this new aspect of your life.

In all honesty, waking up at 4 a.m., whether it is summer or winter, to go to the gym, is one of the hardest things you will ever do. It is not easy and the only way you can do it is through willpower.

Let us unpack the idea of willpower first before we relate it to exercise. We live in a world of immediate gratification. One Instagram video is too boring? No problem, we can just swipe onto the next one. You want food but you don't feel like cooking? No problem, you can get food delivered to your door without even leaving your sofa. Things have become so instantly that as the human race, we have almost forgotten what it is like to work or wait for something. In a world that gives you instant gratification, willpower is the thing that encourages you to wait and work hard for long-term success.

Willpower is having the ability not to give in and succumb to the immediate positive you will experience, but rather working hard and waiting for the ideal moment where you will reap what you have been working so hard toward achieving for the longest time.

Do you know the candy bar that is sitting in your pantry that you have been waiting to devour? Willpower is being able to leave that candy bar in the pantry, day after day, knowing it is there, but also knowing that it is not your cheat day, and it is not going to get you anywhere closer to your goal.

In terms of exercising, willpower is waking up at 4 a.m. and heading to the gym no matter how tired or cold you are. Instant gratification is snoozing your alarm or turning it off and staying in your warm and cozy bed sleeping peacefully. It is comforting, and it is satisfying. But willpower is knowing that you have a goal you would like to reach in six months' time. It is knowing and understanding that six months is a very long time away, but every small step that you take or don't take now will impact how you meet that goal.

It is great to have willpower, we know, the benefits are endless, and you are basically a superior human being. But we need to consider what happens if you don't have any willpower and decide to take on the mammoth undertaking of weight loss. You see, you cannot begin your weight loss journey with just willpower alone. Unfortunately, it is not enough to keep you on track to lose weight, especially maintaining this weight loss because, at some point, you are going to reach your goal—and then what happens? Willpower is just one part of the many components required not just to lose weight but to maintain the results long-term.

On your weight loss journey, you may find the abrupt changes in lifestyle leading to faster weight loss. But eventually, the rate at which you lose weight is going to decrease. It takes a lot of willpower to pursue health and fitness even though you are not guaranteed to see constant results.

When you pursue weight loss and health without any willpower at all, you will likely be faced with crippling difficulties. If you ever wondered why so many people have a long trail of failed diets in their past is because of their lack of willpower which ultimately leads them to seek out quick-fix diets, and not stick to them when the going gets tough. Having no willpower will likely be the biggest roadblock you will face on your weight loss journey because losing weight means being restricted to the things you usually have free access to.

If you take anything away from this book, it will be an understanding of the sheer determination that is required to pursue a healthy lifestyle, not just for now, but forever. The determination and dedication that comes with pursuing this journey cannot be fabricated by just anyone, it cannot be pulled out from thin air, and for the most part, needs to come from within you.

How to Boost Your Willpower

There are some people that I have found myself looking at in absolute awe, having the ability to wake up as soon as their alarm goes off, staying dedicated to their professional "hustle," having the unmatched ability to choose healthy food over junk food, and the ability to stick to an exercise routine almost religiously. These are the people who are worthy of admiration, and I never shy away from complimenting them on their diligence. But when I ask them how they got to this point, the one thing that is certain is that they weren't born with this diligence and willpower. It took hard work and a deep-seated need to no longer live life on a destructive path that led to them building up their willpower.

On the complete opposite end of the spectrum exists the individuals who have little to no willpower. These are the ones who find it hardest to start, let alone stick to the pursuit of weight loss and health. They are the ones who are constantly tempted by the candy in the house, the ones who prefer sleep rather than doing any other task, and those who most people can relate to. What I have found is that those with less willpower are often the ones who haven't had anything severe enough to push them to change their ways. Let me give you an example: I myself became the person I am today because of a health scare and having high cholesterol that pushed me at a young age to reconsider my entire life. Someone who is entirely dedicated to work may know what it is like to not have a job or to lose a job because of a lack of dedication. This usually serves as a turning point that motivates them to strengthen their willpower and pursue the life they hope for.

What if you can build your willpower without facing a catastrophic event that scares you into getting your life straight? Pursuing a healthy lifestyle because you are terrified of your deteriorating health is not enough to keep you on the right track when you do experience some positive changes. In fact, it is all too easy to fall back into your old lifestyle the second you start experiencing positive changes. Here is how you can boost your willpower and self-control:

- The first thing you need to know is that self-control doesn't mean torture. Starving yourself and exercising to a point where you can barely walk or enjoy moments with your family is not something that is worthy of bragging about and is not a great portrayal of your self-control. Self-control also means knowing when to stop and when to give yourself a break. Torturing yourself and making sure that every enjoyable part of life is off-limits is no way to live, but you actually exhibit the best forms of self-control when despite being in the presence of temptation, you know what your goal is, and you are not going to let instant gratification impact the goal you are ultimately working toward.

- It will make it easier for you to practice self-control and willpower if you group together and generalize the things you need to do to lose weight. If you need to be in a calorie deficit but you know that you have a hard time cutting out chocolate entirely, then try to cut down a little bit on everything you eat instead of removing all chocolate from your diet entirely.

- You need to understand what willpower is and what it is not. Willpower is the ability to stay motivated, working toward the result you ultimately desire even if it means enduring some pain or discomfort. Willpower is not cutting yourself from all things that life has to offer and being unkind to yourself if you fail. Willpower is getting back on the horse no matter how many times you fall off.

- While it may seem easier said than done, believing in yourself, setting clear goals, detailing your game plan, and making sure you don't spend too much time being stagnant is a great way of strengthening your willpower. Yes, we can add to that list to avoid temptation and get support, and these are great tools to use when you are establishing your willpower. The true test comes when despite the temptation, you can stand firm.

Finding Your Barriers

Wouldn't it be so easy if all knew exactly what was stopping us from being our best selves in life? We could just zip right in with a pair of scissors, cut out the undesirable parts of ourselves, and walk around as perfect and flawless human beings. But that's not the case. We all have things that stand in the way of us becoming our best selves. The only way I can adequately explain how you can find and remedy your own barriers is if I use myself as an example, entirely unpacking all my vulnerabilities for you, the reader, to realize the experience I am talking from and not just from a superficial inflated sense of self.

There are two things you should know about me: 1) I had almost no willpower when I began my fitness and health journey, and 2) I absolutely hated exercise and physical activity. These were my biggest barriers. And learning what they were and confronting them was not easy. Yes, as humans, we are most critical of ourselves, but we also tend to view ourselves through a lens of "it is not as bad as I may think it is." If we had to take the aspects of ourselves that we are most critical of and place them onto someone else, it would become a point of external fixation. As someone who, in my younger years, was constantly focused on my weight, the first thing I noticed about people that I met for the first time was either how amazing their body was, how similarly, they were shaped to the way I was shaped, or how much larger they were compared to me. The comparison was my ultimate demise. And those were my barriers too.

Many people will complain about failed diets and exercises, and now that we have busted the myths about quick-fix diets, there are other reasons why people fail at their weight loss journey and give up so soon before seeing results.

Why are you at the stage in life you are currently at? Why are you currently in a position where you are seeking weight loss strategies and trying to pursue a healthier lifestyle? Whether it is candy bars, a sedentary lifestyle, or anything else in between, the first thing you need to do is identify your barrier. In myself, and in many of my clients, I have found this to be one of the hardest tasks that anyone can undertake. This requires you to confront the weakest version of yourself, the version of yourself that often leads to your own downfall, and the version of yourself that you may not particularly like. But it is only when you acknowledge and confront this version of yourself that you can remedy the problem at the root.

If you know that your barrier is candy bars, and the reason why you are in your current state of health is that you can't resist the urge to eat the candy that is in the house, then you need to remedy the root cause and remove the thing that is causing your downfall. If you are the one in control of doing the shopping, you have the power to entirely remove the temptation and not buy any candy. Your future self will thank you; you will find the time to work on strengthening your willpower, and you will quickly realize that you can actually live without the one thing you thought you absolutely needed.

Aside from working on your own personal barriers, you could also search your daily routine to figure out if you are facing barriers such as fatigue, discomfort before or after exercise, or underlying medical issues that may be standing in the way of you being a healthier version of yourself.

Chapter 7:

Physical Exercise to Lose Weight

In a Sustained and Steady Way

We don't just want to hop on a bandwagon and try to lose weight as fast as we can, only to gain it all back once we become sick of the dietary constrictions a specific diet gives us. We don't want our options to be limited, and we certainly know that just eating a certain way, without exercising, is not going to do the job for sustained and steady weight loss.

We already know that everyone's body is different, and to get the best out of a weight loss program and exercise, you need to play into your own strengths. But before you can identify your strengths and weaknesses, you need to know what body type you have.

While so many people will talk about their "body type" and they may even call themselves "big boned," not many people are able to break this down for you. It may leave you feeling frustrated, wondering why they get to know what their body type is, but you don't. Allow me to delve into this for you so that you can figure out your body type too.

In every group of friends, there are distinct physical differences that exist. There are the skinny friends who seem to be able to eat everything they get hands on but they don't ever gain weight, there are the friends who seem to live in the gym but their physical stature seems to remain pretty constant, and then there is the heavy set friend who eats next to nothing but somehow still manages to pick up weight. All of these fundamental differences exist in body types, also known as somatotypes.

Knowing your body type goes far deeper than just knowing why you look the way you do and why you may struggle to gain or lose weight, it also goes far deeper than genetics and heredity physical traits, although your body type will be greatly influenced by your genetics. Knowing your body type can actively help you up your fitness levels, gain strength, and even lose weight in a way that is tailor-made for you. It can help you personalize diets and training programs so that you get the best out of it for your particular needs.

The three body types that exist are (Wellnessed, 2011):

- Endomorph, which is identified as a shapely physique. Individuals with this body type will have a larger body frame and more body fat.

- Mesomorph, which is defined as a naturally muscular build. These are the individuals who appear as though they work out constantly, but they really don't.

- Ectomorph, which is a naturally thick and slender frame with little mass and a generally small frame.

Your body type, which is greatly influenced by your genes, will be a great explaining factor for why it seems like you can't seem to adjust your physical appearance despite endless efforts of pursuing a healthy and physically active lifestyle.

No one body type is better than the other, and once you realize what your body type is, you also figure out that it holds certain traits that other body types may not hold. Have you noticed how in a single soccer team, so many players seem to build entirely differently, with some having speed and others having skill as their strengths? Their body types ultimately determine in which position of the field will their strength best be capitalized. So, although they are all soccer players, each one adds a unique value to the team.

How to Determine Your Body Type

There are many ways to figure out your body type such as heading into a lab where precise measurements are taken and according to your structure and how different parts of your body measurements in relation to other parts of your body, as well as your lifestyle, may determine the exact body type you are. You see, while your measurements will give you a great external estimate of the body type you may have, the way your body ultimately processes food and exercise will also give insights into the internal functioning of your body and your body type. This is because body type isn't just about physique and physical appearance, but rather about metabolism and the rate at which your body can break down energy.

The general variables that are used to assess your body type are your metabolism, your frame size, your eating habits, your body type calculator, which is usually done by experts in the fields and professionals, and by reflecting on a past version of yourself. You see, by a certain age, things start slowing down, your metabolism slows, your body changes, your eating habits change, and you are no longer the 20-year-old you once were. Think back to your prime days and remember the habits you had then. This can be a great indicator of the body type you might have if your current body isn't serving as a great indicator.

Different Body Types: An In-Depth Focus

If you look at the **endomorph** body types, these individuals tend to have a slower metabolism. These are the individuals who find themselves gaining weight quite easily, but they struggle to lose this weight, and in many cases, this is what leads to them being slightly overweight (Wellnessed, 2011). However, despite this, they don't just gain weight easily, but they gain muscle and strength easily, too. This means that strength and power sports are likely to be the place where they excel.

Consider that these individuals gain weight quite fast; they may be sensitive to carbohydrates in that if they scoff down too many pizza slices, it may be to their demise, and they may add on a couple of pounds almost immediately. The best kind of diet for an individual with an endomorph body type to follow is one that is low in carbs and high in protein, with a heavy focus on healthy fats. Considering that these individuals are already touched by the scourge of having a slower metabolism, crash diets should be avoided at all costs because this can lead to their metabolism becoming even more sluggish and weighed down than it previously was.

The best exercise for an endomorph to engage in would ideally be cardio, which will not only help them burn fat, but will also help them keep the weight off in the long run. But let's be honest, if you do cardio most days of the week, you are bound to get bored. However, individuals with an endomorph body type can also include high-intensity interval training (HIIT) to increase their endurance and their metabolism. Something else that is great for individuals with this body type to consider is non-exercise activity thermogenesis (NEAT). This is basically your body's way of burning calories without technically engaging in any form of exercise. Things such as walking up the stairs, standing, and parking a little further away from the mall entrance are great ways of unintentionally burning a few extra calories.

The **mesomorph** body type is the individuals who many of us envy, they are the ones who seem to only own two-piece bikinis, and they are usually the people on the front covers of magazines while eating pizza and pasta behind the scenes. These are the individuals who gain muscle with little to no effort, and they are blessed with the genes of having low body fat. This means that it is almost effortless for them to look absolutely ripped, with muscles bulging out from everywhere.

With their metabolism functioning quite efficiently, these are usually the individuals who don't seem to worry too much about their weight, and they tend to gain and lose weight quite easily. They are agile and quick on their feet, and they are blessed with both speed and strength. They usually have a medium-sized frame, and their muscles are easy to notice even though they may not put much effort into bulking their muscles up.

Many may think that the individual who has a mesomorph body type has things easy, and the truth is, to some extent, they do. To have a healthy lifestyle and for their body to be a prime example of this lifestyle, they don't need to adjust their diet other than making sure that they eat balanced meals. They don't need to impose many restrictions on their diets, such as reducing carbs, because their metabolism does the trick rather well.

High-intensity and moderate-intensity workouts will usually do them good and they will find themselves easily burning enough calories to maintain their weight loss progress or maintain their current weight.

We all know of someone who has an **ectomorph** body type. These are the individuals who eat just as much, if not more, than anyone at the table, but you can't help but wonder where all the food goes because they are so tiny built. They have very little fat and muscle, and they have an extremely fast metabolism, which makes it harder for them to gain weight, whether it is fat or muscle mass (Wellnessed, 2011). They are tiny and slenderly built, but they excel at endurance activities.

If you do not have an ectomorph body type and you are reading this, you may find yourself filled with envy toward individuals who do have this body type. You may even find yourself levying a friend that has this body type. But the reality is that being skinny doesn't mean that you are healthy, and that is one of the biggest challenges faced by individuals who have an ectomorph body type. You see, weight gain is the most common way that the human body lets you know you are being unhealthy. Weight gain encourages you to pursue a healthier lifestyle. With this fundamental mechanism highly suppressed, individuals with an ectomorph body type tend to lead very unhealthy lifestyles. They can also have high levels of body fat that is stored but they are unaware of this because their BMI range is within normal expectations. This often means that they face a greater risk of diseases such as insulin resistance, high cholesterol, and high blood pressure, all because they follow an unhealthy lifestyle, but they think they are fine because they don't gain weight (Wellnessed, 2011).

For these individuals to have greater overall health and to have more energy, they are recommended to eat nutrient-dense food, and healthy carbs, and if they are seeking to gain weight, they should snack on healthy foods every three hours to increase their calorie intake (Wellnessed, 2011). For ectomorphs, the best form of physical activity that they can pursue is endurance training coupled with strength training.

While you have been reading through these body types, it may be extremely hard or extremely easy to figure out what kind of body type you have. If, after reading this, you still find yourself struggling to figure out in which box you belong, you can seek help from a physician or a professional trainer and dietician. It is also important to know that sometimes the lines between body types can easily blur and you may find yourself being a combination of two different body types. It is also important to not let your body type entirely deter you or dictate your exact physical activities. If your body type is telling you to do more strength training than cardio but you prefer sports that are cardio-based, that doesn't mean you shouldn't do what you love. You can find ways of accommodating and balancing your physical activities.

Now that you understand your body type, you can now begin working on exercises and diets that will work best for your body type. But since this is a long-term game plan, it is not as simple as jumping headfirst into the first exercise machine you see at the gym. There is a safe starting point that must be taken by anyone and everyone who is pursuing a healthier version of themself.

Your starting point is going to be consulting with a physician before beginning your exercise regimen. The reason for this is that you are going to want to pinpoint and isolate any possible physical conditions you may have that may prevent you from over-exerting yourself. In some cases, if you have excessive muscle weakness, your doctor may want to check that your heart can manage certain exercises and they may recommend that you avoid high-intensity training. Muscle weakness may also lead to the possibility of you being injury prone, so, your doctor may advise you to pursue or avoid certain workouts.

Once you find what works for you and have a few variations of the best exercises for your lifestyle and your body type, it is going to take persistence and willpower to stick to it.

Different Types of Workouts

There are endless resources depicting different exercises and variations of those same exercises that can increase or decrease intensity, but what I have found is that as a beginner, this plethora of information can sometimes be overwhelming. Sometimes, you may find different names and types of exercises thrown at you and you have no idea what each of them means. Well, this is going to serve as a starting point to familiarize you with different types of exercises and different moves within each that you can use in your daily exercise programs and regimens.

Strength Training For Women

Many women see strength training and they want to run for the hills. You are not going to grow any muscles that you don't want to grow, but strength training is a very important part of a healthy lifestyle and an effective weight loss plan. Strength training, cardio, endurance, and everything in between best work in the combination of a balanced routine and a proper exercise schedule. If you find yourself struggling to draft a schedule, once again, pull out a pen and paper, and just the way you did in school, draw up a detailed timetable with specific times carved out for your exercise program.

Here are some of the best strength training exercises you could do:

- Front squat—this is an oldie but a goodie. These exercises show that you don't need to reinvent the wheel or be excessively creative; instead, you just need to stick to what works. A front squat is where you go down like you are about to sit in a chair, but there is no chair. It works a number of leg muscles and your core, and you can throw in some arm weights to make it more intense and include some additional muscle groups. With your feet shoulder length apart, your back straight, and your knee not going over your toe, the squat is a great exercise to include in your daily routine.

- Alternating reverse lunge—with or without added weights, a reverse lunge allows you to step back as deep as you can go, dropping the knee of your back leg as close to the ground as possible with the front leg staying planted firmly on the ground and your knee not going over your toe. Alternate your legs each time and this serves as a great strength training workout.

- Bicep curl—this is probably the most commonly depicted workout, and it is the first thing that comes to mind when you think of heading to the gym. A bicep curl is holding a weight in your hand with your elbow firmly in place on your knee or a bench, and you bring the weight upward toward your chin in a controlled motion. However, maintaining control of this motion is of utmost importance and you can't be flailing or swinging the weight around. Additionally, it is important that you use the weights that are best suited to your current fitness levels. If the weights are too heavy, it can cause more harm than good.

- Sumo Squat—much like a normal squat, you are going down into an almost seat-like position, however, instead of having your feet shoulder-width apart, you are going to have your feet placed widely apart and you are going to lean the top part of your body and your arms down toward the center between your legs, much in the same way as a sumo wrestler would do.

- Curtsey lunge—this lunge is an adaptation of a normal lunge and while you will be doing the same motion with your leg out backward, you are actually going to step backward and in the opposite direction (left leg behind the right leg and vice versa), just as you would do a curtsey.

- Glute bridge—great for toning your rear end, a glute bridge is where you lay flat on your back with your legs bent upwards and you thrust your hips upward toward the air. Ideally, you want your knees to be directly above your heels and a straight diagonal line forming from your knees to your shoulders that are still on the ground. This can be done on counts, or you can hold the position.

- Chest press—much like a bicep curl, this move is a quintessential gym position. Laying on your back with either a weight bar or two weights in either hand, you are going to push from your chest upward toward the sky. You may also be in a sitting position, and you will push the weights forward which lowers the resistance but is still effective in developing your overall strength.

Cardio

Cardio workouts are very intentional rhythmic physical activities that are designed to increase your heart rate. Cardio workouts can be as simple as taking a brisk walk, or they can be more intense like burpees, but either way, they are much needed as part of a balanced physical workout. These are some of the best cardio workouts that you can pursue:

- Inclined walking—walking is pretty straightforward and if you do it often enough, it may not feel like a challenge to you all. A great way to add to the intensity of walking is to add an inclination to it. Walking up a hill or walking up a stepping machine to the gym is a great way to add intensity to the task of just walking.

- Stair climber—the reality is that you don't need a specific stair machine to do the exercise. All you really need is a set of stairs and going up and down these stairs at a gradually increasing pace is bound to up your heart rate.

- Rowing—whether you are on a boat or on the rowing machine at the gym, this provides you with a great full-body workout that gets your arms and your legs involved, getting your heart rate up and making sure you break out into a sweat.

- Assault bike—while not as intimidating as it sounds, the assault bike gives you a cycle workout without actually needing to go outdoors. The assault bike is a stationary bike that allows you to increase resistance, make cycling a bit more challenging, and really make your body work. While a bike ride is a great form of exercise, you can still use an assault bike come rain or shine.

A great way of engaging in cardio is by engaging actively in sports of different types. Sports that get your heart rate beating and that encourage you to use many different parts of your body are great forms of cardio. This can include things like boxing, kickboxing, and even jiu-jitsu. The thing about engaging in these types of sports for exercise is that it comes with multiple benefits. If you are engaging in boxing or jiu-jitsu, you may find yourself gaining basic self-defense skills that may prove to be beneficial in everyday life. Engaging in these kinds of sports usually requires some additional forms of exercise, such as jumping rope or jogging.

Additionally, cardio isn't done without any strength or endurance training. The two are often done hand-in-hand for the best outcome. This means that while you are working out on the stair climber, you could have light weights in your hands which requires you to work out both your arms and your legs. You may even consider adding in a bicep curl with these weights while using the stair climber. You would just have to make sure the weight isn't too heavy for such use.

Lower Body and Abdomen

It has almost become a universal joke that encourages men and women alike not to miss leg day during their gym routine. In some cases, you will find individuals with beautifully sculpted shoulders, backs, and arms, but their legs have little to no muscle definition. But working out your legs is extremely important for more than just aesthetics. You see, some of the largest muscles are located in your legs and thighs. We also know that the more muscle mass you have, the easier it is for your body to lose fat. Therefore, exercising these large muscle groups is a great contributor to losing weight.

However, when you are doing leg exercises, an important part of maintaining balance is to do core exercises as well. This means that you are going to be working your abdomen muscles and your upper legs in similar motions. Lower body and abdominal exercises that you can engage in are:

- Lying leg raises—laying flat on your back, you are going to keep your legs straight and extended and lift them up to the sky. Because you are doing this as a controlled motion, you are not going to be relying on momentum to raise your legs. This means that through the work of your ab muscles, as well as the work of your leg muscles, you will be raising your legs, making sure to target and work out that particular part of your body.

- Leg in and out—sitting on your bum, leaning back on your hands, extending and contracting your legs toward your abdomen and out again. This will work out your abdominal muscles and it will provide endurance training for your leg muscles.

- Scissor kicks—much like the lying leg raises, the scissor kick exercises use the same concept, but you will be alternating the legs that go up into the sky, and instead of a large range of motion, you are going to make smaller movements which require greater control.

- Crunches—this is some people's worst nightmare, but it is a great exercise for directly working out your abdominal muscles. Crunches target specific abdominal sections whereas sit-ups target all abdominal muscles. While these exercises are great for weight loss, it is important to know that you can build your abs beneath the fat around your abdomen. It is therefore important to remember that you may not see any definition, but you will most likely see a difference once you lose fat around your waist.

Each individual type of exercise serves its own purpose. It is important that you don't focus on one type of exercise and neglect the others because the best way to achieve the best body for yourself is to use a combination of all these exercises. Each will fulfill its purpose within your body, and you won't look like someone who misses leg day.

You may find that your muscles are sore and achy, and you don't want to work out the same muscle groups tomorrow that you worked out today. This is good, and it is important that you don't overexert your muscles. You see, when you feel the ache in your muscles after an intense workout, that is a sign that your muscles are growing. In order to grow, some tissues may have to tear and repair themselves. In moderation, this is good, and it means growth. If it happens excessively, it leads to injury. Once you feel the burn and the ache, you can avoid working out the same muscle groups the next day so that you give your muscles time to repair. If you are planning a workout routine, I always recommend that my clients choose one day in the week to focus on a particular body part, which means it gives them about a week for their muscles to repair before they push themselves again. So, let every Monday be leg day, let every Tuesday be biceps, and every Wednesday be back, or something similar. This means that you give your muscles time to heal while remaining quite consistent in your training.

And just like that, you begin sculpting the body of your dreams.

Chapter 8:

Figuring Out the Dietary Plans for

Weight Loss

Eating. Why does it have to be so complicated? In a perfect world, chocolate would be a salad and we'd all be skinny and healthy. Unfortunately, that is not the case. The world has been infiltrated by unhealthy foods, deep fried and covered in sugar. We have been tossed into the lifestyle of being excessively busy, not having time to cook a healthy meal, being forced to choose between speed and convenience, and health, but not many other options since we can't compromise other aspects of our lives.

While it may seem like being caught in a humorous cycle, when you are actually the one at the center of this cycle trying to get your health on track, it can be extremely overwhelming and can be a great source of anxiety. It may seem like every move and every effort you make at becoming healthier; something stands in your way.

I know that feeling all too well. There were many instances where I would know exactly what I was making for dinner, my whole family was going to enjoy a hearty and healthy meal, but there was a pile-up on the highway that caused an hour delay which meant I needed to stop to buy an often unhealthy yet quick meal for my family and me. These setbacks didn't happen when I was far along in my health and weight loss journey. Instead, they happened when I was just embarking on this journey, making everything harder than necessary from the onset of my attempts to live a healthier life.

So how do you solve this seemingly never-ending problem? Life is always going to happen, and while there might not be anything standing in your way every day, there are many days when cooking a healthy meal just doesn't seem feasible. The best solution for these moments is meal prep.

I know you have heard of meal prep before and how great it is, and you probably thought the same thing that I thought when I was first introduced to meal prep: "I don't want to spend my weekend cooking for the whole week." But let me assure you that your future self will be so happy.

Aside from taking out the inconvenience of buying takeout when you are running late, meal prep provides you with mental benefits too. It reduces your decision fatigue, taking the guesswork out of this one simple task and allowing you to know exactly what is going on in your body.

You have probably seen the videos on social media and looked at people organizing their pantries and preparing meals for their families for the week. And while it may seem achievable, it is great for anyone who is hoping to pursue a healthier lifestyle. Meal prep isn't about spending your entire weekend cooking. Instead, it is about investing a little bit of extra time to prepare healthy food and gaining that time through the week. I found myself very concerned about doing meal prep because I thought that in an attempt to spend more time with my family after work; I am actually taking time away from them during the weekend. It felt like I wasn't winning either way. And then I made it a family activity and let me tell you, meal prep is not only great for our minds and bodies, but for our hearts and our familial relationships too.

Meal prep isn't about cooking more or buying more groceries; instead, I found batch cooking and prepping my ingredients ahead of time is the best way to save time. Batch cooking basically means cooking entire meals, dishing them out into containers that are ready to be eaten, and just taking them out and warming them as is on the day we're meant to eat them. This meant that I had little to no work to do on days when I ran late or when we had to attend any form of school function in the evening.

Ingredient prep was for the days when I wanted to feel like I was on vacation when I came home from work. If I needed chicken to be marinated or vegetables to be cut, I would prep these vegetables over the weekend. In most cases, even if I came home from work at my normal time, I could throw all the ready-prepped ingredients into a pot and forget about it until it was ready. This left me with the opportunity to spend time with my kids, watching TV or playing board games instead of chopping raw ingredients in the kitchen.

Different Types of Dietary Methods

Now that you know how to meal prep, it is time to figure out *what* to prepare. Before we delve into the different types of dietary methods that exist when you are pursuing weight loss, there is something important that I have to draw your attention to. We have already established that this journey is going to be anything but easy. We also know that you have to create a weight loss plan that works for *you*. This means that what you eat is probably going to be different from what the rest of your family eats. If you are the person who cooks at home, this may seem like yet another burden to bear. But the reality is that it is entirely worth it when you consider that you are changing your lifestyle for the better. Yes, changing your family's eating habits and setting them on the path to a healthier lifestyle is going to be extremely beneficial, but if you are deciding to strictly follow a specific eating plan, you may want to consider being a little less strict with your family which means adjusting the quantities that you cook, or if you are having a carb-free day, you may need to consider cooking carbs for them.

Intermittent Fasting

The first type of dietary method that you could pursue weight loss is intermittent fasting. The concept of fasting is often deeply rooted in religious practices as a way of sanctifying the body and cleansing the body. In religious practices, fasting also serves as a sacrifice, a payment of sorts that one is willing to make in return for purity and answered prayers.

Many people find themselves experiencing multiple health benefits through religious fasting and this has led to the concept of an intermittent fast. You see, fasting with a religious purpose in mind cannot be sustained for the long term for two reasons. The first reason is that if you fast the way you did with a spiritual intention every day, you may lose touch with the spiritual basis for your fasting and your intentions may become distorted. Also, some people are not religious or spiritual and there may not be an initial driving force to get them to consider fasting at all. Secondly, many people fast for different durations and with different intensities during religious practices. Some religions require followers to fast from sunrise to sunset, others require fasting to be abstaining only from meat or certain types of foods, and other religions may pursue fasts that last more than one consecutive day and that only permit you to drink water. Each type of fasting is different and may not be sustainable in the long term. The best solution for this is intermittent fasting.

Intermittent fasting, while not a religious practice, allows you to experience the physical benefits that come with fasting while being realistic for you to pursue it on a long-term basis.

Intermittent fasting allows you to fast for a certain period within 24 hours a day, and it allows you a window period in your day to eat and snack. The benefits of fasting provide you with the ability to begin self-regulating your blood sugar and blood pressure, but it doesn't mean that during the period where you are allowed to eat on your day, you can eat any food. You still need to plan what healthy meals your body type needs to eat. This can be made up of protein meals and high-protein snacks.

Keto Diet

Another beneficial eating method for weight loss is the ketogenic diet, also known as the keto diet. A keto diet consists of a high-fat diet, medium protein intake, and low carbs. It will include things like substituting rice for cauliflower and focusing on eating eggs, avocados, and other healthy fats.

However, as with any other diet plan, you need to follow this diet with caution. If you suffer from high cholesterol, following a high-fat diet may negatively contribute to your cholesterol levels, especially if you are not careful about the types of fats that you are consuming. It is for that reason that you consult with your physician before undertaking any dietary restrictions.

Inducing Weight Loss Through Food Elements

There are general changes that you can make to your diet that will ultimately boost weight loss in your body. Things such as drinking more water, eating more protein, taking in more fiber, and adding a variety of food groups into your diet will induce weight loss, especially if this will be a change to your existing diet. Your body will ultimately process these new foods differently and will allow you to lose weight on its own.

The Impact of a Proper Dietary Plan In Your Daily Life

Following a dietary plan is not just about losing weight or finding an eating plan that will help you shed pounds. While that may be a primary goal, it is extremely important to consider what you are eating and make sure that you get enough of all food groups so that your body doesn't become malnourished in any way. While you may be eating potato fries on a daily basis, you may find yourself facing an iron deficiency because you aren't taking in leafy vegetables. So, while your belly is full, you may still be malnourished.

Having a proper diet not only feeds your body but also feeds your mind and your emotions. It also adds to healthy growth, and while you may think that you aren't going to grow anymore, it keeps you healthy and functional even though you aren't growing anymore. Healthy nutrition that comes from a healthy eating lifestyle leads to great overall health and well-being. You will find your mental acuity is higher than before, and you may even find yourself smiling more often.

Despite the importance of having a proper dietary plan in place, many people make some common mistakes, and they don't even realize just how severe these mistakes can be for their overall health. Here are some common mistakes that people make when it comes to their diet and by being aware of this, you can make a conscious effort to try to avoid these mistakes.

- The first mistake that people make is skipping breakfast. I have had people ask me why breakfast is such a big deal because they had avoided breakfast and actually lost weight. I know it sounds great but skipping breakfast can disrupt your blood sugar levels and the control you have of your blood sugar which leads to unnecessary sugar spikes and you feeling slow and sluggish when you do eventually eat. Skipping breakfast can often lead to people eating high-calorie snacks and they often do this unconsciously. We have all been there where we were so hungry that we quickly ate two packets of chips and forgot about those snacks soon after. Eating breakfast minimizes this form of unhealthy eating.

- Just as we forget that we have eaten two bags of chips, we also forget a lot of the other small snacks that we eat during the day. Small pieces of candy here and there, juice and sodas, and other high-calorie snacks that we often take in quantity rather than quality are easily forgotten. I usually remedy this by making a note of everything I eat throughout the day. While this may seem tedious at first, it allows you to be more conscious and aware of what you are eating on a daily basis.

- On the other end of the spectrum, it is a common misconception that snacking entirely is a bad idea. However, if you snack on the right foods, you actually do your body a world of good. Your body doesn't get very hungry and stores fats, and you may find your metabolism speeding up. It is important that your snacks are high in protein and low in calories.

- People often make a mistake between low-fat and low-calorie. Perhaps you have also fallen victim to this, and you stock up on low-fat snacks and foods, forgetting that you are still putting a high number of calories into your body. This ultimately slows down your weight loss and despite the low-fat foods you are eating, you may even find yourself gaining weight.

- Many people forget about what they sip on. You see, water is essential for weight loss because it speeds up your metabolism, but also, drinking juice and sodas, and meal replacement shakes are full of calories that we often forget to count. So, you may be wondering why all you eat is salad and yet you aren't losing weight, but you keep ordering a milkshake or a high-calorie and high-fat coffee that adds to the calories you are consuming.

- Lastly, many people think they are doing their body favors by cutting out specific food groups, and often, the food group that people cut out is dairy. What they don't realize is that dairy contains a lot of calcium and calcium is needed to burn fat. In actual fact, your body tends to produce more fat when it is deprived of calcium, so cutting out dairy may not be the best solution for weight loss, just as long as you count the calories you are taking in with that glass of milk or the extra slice of cheese you are having (Ratini, 2022).

Dieting Is Not About Eating Less

The concept of quality over quantity is most prevalent in food and the type of food people eat. You see, dieting is not just about eating less. When people cut down the quantity of food they eat and they try to eat less, they don't really do it in a controlled way. They don't cut down on food while still maintaining a balanced diet which often leads to losing out on important nutrients.

We may have all made this mistake before—we have decided to eat less and so we choose to cut out all carbs, even the carbs that are considered good for us. This ultimately leads to a deficiency in the nutrients and all the good things that these healthy carbs provide us with.

So, when you are pursuing a diet or an eating plan, my recommendation is not to eat less, but to eat in a controlled way. This allows you to get everything your body needs while reducing the number of calories you take in. You are not losing out on any one specific thing, but rather, you are getting everything you need in smaller quantities.

Selective eating and portion control each come with their own pitfalls, and it is up to you to decipher what adds to and what takes away from your overall health. But this often stems from a lack of knowledge or understanding about what benefits different foods provide to your body. I know it might seem overwhelming and it may seem like you need to be a diet expert to know and understand what types of foods you should eat. And when it does feel overwhelming, you can rest assured knowing that there are people out there who have dedicated their careers to coaching and assisting individuals on their weight loss and health journey, making sure that they lose weight in a healthy way and that they sustain this weight loss.

It is easy for me to tell you to eat specific food groups because it is beneficial for specific reasons and bodily functions. But the reality is that if you truly want to understand why certain foods are needed, you need to consult with a physician and a nutritionist. They will provide you with a deep insight and understanding of the importance of a proper diet, not just understanding why your body needs it but also understanding how your body breaks down each type of food that it needs.

Chapter 9:

All You Need To Know About

Intermittent Fasting

If you haven't heard of intermittent fasting before, it can seem a bit overwhelming. Thinking about staying away from food for excessively long periods of time may make you light-headed. But the reality is, it has gained immense popularity in recent years as an effective means of weight loss. Not only is it effective, but it can be done long term as an effective way of maintaining your body.

So, what exactly is intermittent fasting? We already know that it has been a foundational pillar in many religious practices, and we know that fasting is the concept of abstaining from food. But when it comes to dieting and health, intermittent fasting is not so much to do with what you eat, but rather about *when* you eat (Johns Hopkins Medicine, n.d.).

Intermittent fasting is not a diet, but rather an eating routine. Now, while the focus isn't so much on what you eat but rather on when you eat, it is still important to be conscious and aware of what you eat. Intermittent fasting isn't about following this strict pattern and routine but scoffing down junk food when you do actually eat.

Let's unpack this. Intermittent fasting is giving yourself a period of the day when you are fasting and not taking in any food, and a window period when you can eat. You basically schedule your meals so that you get the most energy usage and expenditure out of what you put into your body.

Ideally, during intermittent fasting, you will be eating during the times of your day when you are burning the most calories. There are different types of intermittent fasting options that you can pursue, which will be discussed later in this chapter, but let me give you a brief insight into how this works. For example, you may decide to fast for 16 hours in your day, and you may decide that your eating window period will be eight hours in the day. This may seem like a long time to not be eating, but when you consider that your fasting period can also include the eight hours you spend sleeping, it makes it much easier. Many people opt to start their eating window period at around 11 a.m. which means that they are allowed to eat their daily calorie intake between 11 a.m. and 7 p.m., which includes breakfast, lunch, dinner, and all the snacks they intend on eating in a day.

With meals scheduled closer together, you may automatically find yourself eating smaller portions which are great to reduce your calorie intake, and in these eight hours, you can focus on what it is you are putting in your body. Because you are not decreasing your calorie intake, you find yourself maintaining muscle mass while losing fat.

This may raise some concerns and seem counterproductive in that you are not eating breakfast, which is something that we are always told not to do when we are on a weight loss journey, but technically, you are not missing breakfast, you are just eating it later in the day. Additionally, if this seems like a deal breaker, you may consider starting your eating window period at 8 a.m. and closing that window at 4 p.m.

This strategy is great for fat loss and can be done for long periods of time. In fact, when many people begin intermittent fasting, they tend to stick to it permanently. Modern society has falsely given us the idea that we need to eat three meals a day. The reality is that, as long as we are taking in enough water, humans can successfully fast for days at a time. Now, this is not what you need to do during intermittent fasting, but when you consider that in ancient times humans were hunters and gatherers, it is easy to realize that they probably had to go long periods of time without food. They did this successfully.

Our current lifestyle has become progressively worse over time as technology, computer-based jobs, effortless streaming, and unhealthy sleeping patterns have come into existence. This means that we spend more time being inactive and eating unhealthily than we used to before.

So, what is the science behind intermittent fasting and how does it actually work? Well, When you are not eating for a prolonged period of time, even within a 24-hour period, your body does something called metabolic switching which is when it burns all its sugar stores and starts burning fats (Johns Hopkins Medicine, n.d.). But because you are not doing this for an excessive period and you are doing it quite consistently, your body knows that it doesn't need to hold on to fat stores to avoid starvation because your body is constantly being fed. This makes your body quite comfortable with expanding its excess fat.

You see, when your body is in a fed state, which is the period from when you start eating and ends three to five hours after you eat, your body absorbs and digests the food you have just eaten. However, during this fed state, your body finds it extremely difficult to burn fat. This is because your insulin levels are extremely high. Thereafter, your body is no longer actively digesting a meal, and if you choose to fast in that time, this stage of not actually digesting a meal can last up to 12 hours, which makes it easier for your body to burn fat because your insulin levels are at a constant low (Clear, 2012).

So, let us look at this as a practical application. If you follow the "normal" way of life eating three meals a day, you will be filling your body with food even before it reaches the stage where it is no longer actively digesting food. This means that your body has less time to burn fat. However, during intermittent fasting, your body has up to 16 hours to burn fat.

Benefits of Intermittent Fasting

If you haven't already noticed the benefits of intermittent fasting, let us delve a bit deeper into it. One of the greatest benefits of intermittent fasting is that it really takes a lot of the thought out of when and what to eat in your day. Intermittent fasting is about slightly changing and adapting your lifestyle, so whether you find yourself eating three smaller meals during your eating period, or whether you are eating two meals, you have less to worry about when it comes to meal prep.

Intermittent fasting can also increase your lifespan, it may reduce your risks of cancer (although research is sparse), it is easier to stick to than dieting, and it may even help your body maintain and balance its blood sugar and insulin levels.

When you consider that it is healthier and easier than dieting and that it is safe to pursue long-term as a lifestyle, intermittent fasting really does appear to be a winner.

Intermittent fasting also directly contributes to removing excess belly fat, which is extremely beneficial for women who are meant to have some fat around their bellies, but not excessive amounts. Lastly, the psychological benefits that come with intermittent fasting work hand-in-hand with the physical benefits. You may find yourself having a clearer mind, having greater concentration, and not feeling as slow or sluggish as you would normally after eating a big meal.

Types of Intermittent Fasting Plans

Ideally, most of us want to engage in practices that don't require us to change our current lifestyles too much. As humans, we are not fans of change. So, when you are hoping to add intermittent fasting into your lifestyle, the great thing is that it is adaptable. There are a number of intermittent fasting programs that you could use which may fit into your lifestyle more easily. If you are a morning person and you enjoy eating breakfast earlier, you can adjust your fasting accordingly; if supper is an event in your home, you could make sure that your intermittent fasting doesn't prevent you from engaging in family dinner traditions with your family.

The first method that you could choose is the 16:8 fasting method which is where, as previously mentioned, you would fast for 16 hours and eat for eight hours in the day. Much like this method, there is an 18:6 fasting method that allows you to eat for six hours in the day and fast for 18 hours in the day. You could ultimately decide the time that your eating window will start, and it is important to know that sleeping is counted in your fasting period.

Next, you have the 5:2 approach which requires you to eat normally for five days of the week, and for two days in the week, you eat an extremely low-calorie diet. Your calorie intake on your "fasting" days would be no higher than 500–600 calories on those days (Johns Hopkins Medicine, n.d.).

There are also options where you can choose to fast for an entire 24-hour period in a week or you could fast every alternative day. Ideally, the option you choose would be most beneficial to your current lifestyle and that would most effortlessly fit into your current lifestyle.

Foods To Eat During Intermittent Fasting

Now that we have the concept of time sorted out, which is the most important aspect of intermittent fasting, it is important to figure out what you should be eating during your editing periods. Firstly, let us look at what you can't have during your fasting period.

During your fasting period, while you may not be able to take in any foods that will cause your body to go into digestion mode and cause your insulin to spike, it is important to make sure you are properly hydrated, which means water is a must. Additionally, you may also consider taking in some tea or coffee, if you are a tea or coffee drinker.

When you are in your eating period, it is not an opportunity to eat anything and everything. Do not allow yourself to fall into the misconception that you can eat an unhealthy meal and your body will burn it off during your fasting period. Instead, You need to make sure that you are eating foods with high-quality fats which include fats from avocados and nuts, that you should be taking in lean protein and vegetable protein, and you need to be conscious about your gut health making sure to take in the right amounts of fiber, coupled with carbohydrates that are sufficient to sustain your body during the fasting period of a day.

Next, you need to schedule the meals that you will eat during your eating period. If we again use the 16:8 method as an example, and you consider setting your eating window between 11 a.m. and 7 p.m., You may consider skipping breakfast in the regular sense of the word and having your first meal at 11 a.m. which can consist of a breakfast meal, or it can be something entirely different and creative. What I like to recommend that my clients do is make sure this meal contains fiber, protein, healthy carbs, and fats, which often come in the form of a sandwich because this is a great option for when you are probably already at work. If you do have the opportunity to be eating cereal or eggs and toast, then take that opportunity too.

Snacking is important for weight loss. No, you didn't read wrong, and your eyes have not deceived you. But the truth is that high-protein snacks are actually extremely important for weight loss. Even when you are in a calorie deficit you want to make sure you are taking in enough calories to achieve and maintain a healthy weight loss. This means actively incorporating snacks, in a healthy way, into your food intake. You can then choose to have your last meal for the day at around 6 p.m. and have a light snack an hour later, giving your body enough time to actively digest your food before you sleep.

Now, we already know that food is not the only thing that contributes to weight loss and weight management, but it has to be done in tandem with exercise, as well. This is no different if you are intermittent fasting. However, what does need attention is how and when you exercise.

The best time to exercise during intermittent fasting is early in the day. This allows you to capitalize on the natural energy your body may have. Ideally, outside of intermittent fasting, working out needs to happen between meals so that you have enough fuel to exercise, and so that you don't feel depleted after a workout. The same can be done during intermittent fasting, but if that is not a reasonable possibility for you, then exercising as early in the day as possible is best for you.

Whether you are considering intermittent fasting or not, it is not anything to be tied down by and it is not the do-or-die option for sustained weight loss. In the next chapter, we will delve deeper into a keto diet as a possible dietary method for weight loss.

Chapter 10:

All You Need To Know About Keto

Diet

You may or may not have heard of a ketogenic diet, and you may wonder if this is a long-term approach to weight loss or if it is just another fad that you can hop on the bandwagon and enjoy losing a few pounds. But a keto diet is an extremely effective means to achieve weight loss, and ultimately increase your overall health.

A keto diet is a low-carb, high-fat diet that requires you to make substantial lifestyle changes if you haven't already been following this diet for a while. Basically, the foods that you eat need to have the highest percentage of *healthy* fat, a moderate intake of protein, and extremely few carbs.

Now, how does this translate into weight loss if you are going to be consuming a diet that is made up predominantly of fats? Well, before I answer your question, it is important to know that you are going to be focused on consuming healthy fats. This means fish, nuts, avos, and healthy oils, instead of chocolate and chocolate spreads.

The way a ketogenic diet works is that it functions on a hormonal and a molecular level. The food that you put into your body ultimately manipulates the way your body processes foods, the hormones it releases, and how you burn your energy. At a physiological level, your body experiences a change.

When you take on a keto diet, your body decreases the amount of appetite-enhancing hormones that it may produce when you take in fewer carbohydrates. Insulin levels are lower which means you get fuller faster, and you may find yourself not really craving something sweet after a big and heavy meal. On the keto diet, your body's main fuel source becomes ketone, which is what reduces hunger in the body. This ultimately leads to your body burning more calories because your metabolic rate increases as you are converting fat and protein into glucose for fuel rather than carbs.

For weight loss, the keto diet has been proven to be beneficial, but it is not without flaws. The bottom line of the keto diet is that it is still a diet. This means that it may not be effective in the long term and may lead to a number of health factors because of the lack of carbs and high levels of protein and fat that you are required to consume. Unlike intermittent fasting which can be done in the long term, a keto diet is not viable for prolonged periods of time.

Since your body is deprived of glucose, you may actually find yourself facing some strange side effects from the keto diet. Because of the drastic change in your diet, especially if you were someone who had a particular inclination toward bread and other carbs, you may find yourself feeling light-headed, having severe leg and muscle cramps, facing digestive issues, and even having irregular menstrual periods. You may also find this extreme change in diet to cause bad breath and a decrease in your bone density.

You may also experience the keto flu which is what happens when your body begins burning ketones instead of glucose for energy. This is the active fat-burning process of the keto diet, but the adjustment can be brutal on the body leading to extreme flu-like symptoms including headaches, weakness, vomiting, and nausea (The Healthline Editorial Team, 2018).

The Basic Principles of the Ketogenic Diet

The keto diet really is all about balance and consistency. You will be balancing the meal ratio with exercise to get the most effective fat-burning solution for your body. But it is important to know that what you choose to eat, the meals you choose to put into your body, and the type of fat that you choose to put into your body needs to be healthy.

If you are putting the wrong types of fats into your body, then weight loss may not be as attainable. Additionally, the keto diet is one that you need to consult with a doctor or a medical expert before you consider pursuing it. The reason for this is that a high-fat diet may not be suitable for you if you have underlying medical conditions such as heart problems, gout, and high cholesterol. It is therefore important that you consult with a doctor, do the necessary blood tests, and make sure that your body is healthy before pursuing the keto diet.

Quick and Easy Meal Ideas for Keto

If you decide, after medical consultation, that the keto diet is the best way for you to begin your weight loss journey or to see the most effective results, then you obviously need to know what foods and meals you should prepare to get the most effective results from this diet. I can tell you now that chocolate is not going to be a very high part of this diet. You also need to know that a keto diet is quite strict, and you need to adhere to it quite strictly if you hope to reap the rewards of this diet.

So as a beginner to the keto diet, it can seem overwhelming not knowing what to eat and you may feel extremely restricted, however, there are ways to introduce variety to your diet so that you don't get bored of the food. Ultimately, even through this eating plan, you don't want to get bored or tired with what you are eating.

Breakfast Foods and Smoothies

Smoothies are great, everyone loves them, and they make great breakfasts and lunches. They are versatile and can be eaten as a part of almost every meal. Some of the best smoothies that you could consider are berry and avo smoothies or almond butter smoothies. All you will need is to add ingredients such as mixed berries, avo slices, milk, and some honey, if need be, throw it into a blender with some ice, if you so choose, and have it for breakfast or lunch. For your almond butter smoothie, you can add almond butter, honey, bananas, and milk to your blender with ice if you so choose and have that as a great breakfast.

When you think of breakfast foods, the first thing that probably comes to mind is eggs. Eggs are perfect for keto diets because they are packed with protein and fat. Adding extra protein and fatty foods to your eggs can definitely help. This is where you can consider making pulled pork frittata or spinach and feta cheese omelet. Cooked with a bit of avocado oil or olive oil is sure to make this your best keto breakfast food yet.

When you consider that fish has a number of healthy fats in it, it is almost like a keto superfood. You could consider having a salmon and cream cheese roll-up that has cucumbers and is perfectly spiced. This not only makes a great breakfast meal, but it also makes a great lunch or dinner meal, and after all, isn't convenience what we're looking for?

Sausages, scrambled eggs, bacon, and a variety of cheeses form the best part of any keto breakfast. You can try mixing and matching these foods and you are guaranteed to have a great breakfast every day, it won't even feel like you are on a diet.

Salads and Soups

Throwing some variation into the mix, you could make a creamy tomato and basil soup, broccoli and cheese soup, or coconut and cauliflower shrimp soup which will have all the elements you need for a successful keto diet. The great thing about cooking soups when you are on the keto diet is that you are guaranteed to have leftovers. Do you know what this means? Life will be easier, and you get to live with the blissful convenience of having lunch the next day already planned. Soups are great for freezing and you can eat them on alternate days, so you don't get tired of eating the same thing over and over again.

Salads on a keto diet are not the same as the salads you would think of. No iceberg lettuce, cucumbers, and some tomatoes for color. Instead, you get to have tasty and delicious salads that taste like a piece of heaven. You can make a Mexican egg salad that has eggs, corn, peppers, scallions, garlic, celery, and a lot of seasoning in it to make a delicious side dish or main meal. This is great for a BBQ, and it makes a great dinner time or lunchtime meal.

Additionally, you could make avocado egg salads which have more traditional salad elements such as lettuce, and it makes for a great meal.

Snacks and Side Dishes

From buttery mushrooms, baked zucchini, cauliflower mashed potatoes, and keto bread, there is rarely an appetizer or meal that won't be made extra delicious without a side dish.

Carb Replacements

Since the very nature of the keto diet is to take in as little carbohydrates as possible, there are many carb alternatives or substitutes that you can use. First, instead of sugar, you can use xylitol or stevia. Second, you can substitute carbs in your meals. For example, instead of rice, you could blend a head of cauliflower roughly, cook it in a few drops of vegetable or olive oil, and have it as a rice substitute. You could also use zucchini spaghetti as a replacement for regular spaghetti and you could use zucchini in place of potato chips. You could also use almond flour in place of normal flour. Feeling for a tortilla wrap? You could use lettuce instead and substantially reduce the number of calories you take in. Something we also tend to forget in our calorie count or as a contributor to carbs is milk, but if you swap it out for almond milk or oat milk, you dramatically reduce the amounts of carbs you take in.

Many people think that the keto diet is the most delicious of all diets. And it probably is true. But when you are eating a high-fat and extremely delicious meal, it is easy to overdo it. It is important during this diet to be extremely conscious and aware of your portion size and to count your calories, so you don't end up putting in more than you are putting out. Ultimately, you want to maintain balance as much as possible.

Chapter 11:

The Psychological Aspect of

Weight Loss for Women

Why is psychology such an important part of weight loss? We know that we need our minds to do anything that will yield a physical manifestation, but is there more to the mind and psyche when it comes to weight loss than we previously thought? The reality is that while we do need strong minds to lose weight, we need our minds to be even stronger to keep the weight off. Many studies have found that people gain back the weight they have lost from diets within three to five years of losing the weight, sometimes even sooner (UCI Health, 2020).

As important as your physical health is, and as much as you are going to be eating right and working out, all of those efforts are futile if you don't exercise your mind. Mental exercise is just as important as physical exercise. But how do you get yourself into the mental space that you need to be in for weight loss? Well, you are going to start by doing a mental evaluation of yourself. Now, don't get me wrong, this is not going to be a psych assessment that is going to determine if you should be in a mental institute, but it is rather going to be an assessment of where your mental well-being currently is and how where you are currently may affect your weight loss.

When you are beginning to plan your weight loss journey, you are going to first do your psyche assessment to see where you are, and then you are going to see what mental blocks you are facing that may be standing in your way of achieving physical health.

Let us start with the psychological assessment you are going to do on yourself (Institute for the Psychology of Eating, 2018):

- The first thing you need to evaluate is your stress levels. Stress, whether it is a deadline or not, or us being unhappy with our current state of life and feeling like we may never get past it, can all affect our ability to lose weight. Your body goes into survival mode and at a metabolic and physiological level, it is harder for you to burn fat. So, when you begin efforts to lose weight, you need to look at the stressors in your life and begin working on treating those at the root so that your weight loss journey has a higher chance of being successful.

- You then need to assess your pleasure. Pleasure also contributes to weight loss, and you need to make sure that you are enjoying your weight loss efforts. If you aren't, you may find yourself unsuccessful in your weight loss attempts. Finding the pleasure and joy in weight loss and in health will make the entire journey much easier and it will make it easier to see results.

- Our behavior is a physical manifestation of our psychology. When you make a conscious effort and tally your behavior, you quickly realize that this ultimately will affect our success in our health. The little things we do will either contribute to or take away from our efforts of losing weight. So, take a look at your behaviors—do you like to just sit on the couch and do nothing after eating a big meal or do you prefer to take a brisk walk after your meals? Do you find yourself eating dessert every day? Do you drink enough water? Are you entirely aware of how much you fill your plate? All of these behavioral aspects need to be considered when you are carrying out your psychological assessment of yourself, and the answers you will make will impact your success in your weight loss journey.

Next, you need to look at the things that may serve as possible blockages in your weight loss journey. I am not talking about the almost unrealistic blockage of having a pantry full of candy and nothing else to eat (and a part of me admits this seems like a dream rather than a blockage), but rather about the mental blockages that almost lead to us standing in our own way in our weight loss journey.

These are some of the most common psychological blocks that many people face on their weight loss journey (Frey, 2021):

- Having an all-or-nothing approach to weight loss may seem like something to strive toward, but it is actually a distorted way of thinking. This causes people to have unrealistic expectations and if they do fail on their weight loss journey, the downfall is catastrophic. Living on two ends of the extreme in this all-or-nothing approach is a way of negatively impacting your success. Yes, when you do experience success, it will be high, but your failures will make you feel down and out more than anything.

- Having a negative body image can stop your success before you even start. A negative image doesn't mean ignoring the signs of an unhealthy lifestyle. You can look at yourself in the mirror, and realize you need to lose weight, while still loving yourself and what you see in the mirror. You just need to learn to love the potential version of yourself too.

- Stress and depression are mental disorders that have physical manifestations. It is important to overcome these blocks so that you can clear your mind about the challenges you will inevitably face during your weight loss journey. We know that weight loss isn't easy, and stress and depression make it all too easy to fall off the wagon.

There are ways to overcome these blocks during your weight loss journey. The first point is being mindful. Living in the moment and being aware of everything you do and say to yourself is the best starting point you can give yourself. Making small changes in your life, paying close attention to your self-talk, being intentional about your sleeping habits, and actively seeking help when you feel the need, are all ways to help yourself get over these mental blocks in weight loss.

A sound body lives in a sound mind, so you need to start with your mind first to ensure your physical success.

Your Beliefs and Thoughts About Weight Loss

There are common myths that we believe and that we cling to when it comes to weight loss, many of which greatly impact our own way of approaching our health journey. But we need to realize that we are an entirely separate entity from the myths that exist around weight loss. When these myths affect our beliefs and our approach to weight loss is when it becomes our own personal superstitions, and those are the things we need to overcome to get past the blocks we ultimately create for ourselves.

When your state of mind is in the right place you will find yourself losing the right amount of weight that lines up with your psychological state and well-being. And here is where the practice of mindfulness becomes so important. You see, having your mind and body line up usually leads to the healthiest version of yourself that exists. If you lean too far in either direction is where you actually find people lying on two extremes of the spectrum. You get people who are excessively obese and people who suffer from eating disorders such as anorexia nervosa. In these cases, you will find that their minds and their psychology have leaned too far in the wrong direction and that is why they face the challenges that they have.

For weight loss and for weight gain, the best way to achieve either is through mindful practices. Mindfulness keeps you actively aware of your current state and what you are currently doing to enhance or hinder your current state. When you are mindful, you are alert to what you are putting into your body, you fully immerse yourself into workouts, and you learn not to dread the workouts you once hated. This is because you actively feel the discomfort and pain that a workout may cause you, and because you are mindful, you experience the pleasure that comes once you have completed your workout.

A State of Mind

So, we have looked at mental and physical health, but it would be remiss if I did not look at the spiritual state of mind that exists in weight loss. I know it may not seem like spirituality plays a role in weight loss, but when you consider that your body houses a soul, and even if you aren't of that belief and you believe that we go back to the earth after our demise, it is important to take care of whatever power we believe our body houses.

Because we are on a journey to overall and holistic good health, it means taking care of your mind, body, and your soul. With that being said, the last aspect is the soul. When you are healthy physically and mentally, you may find spiritual health following suit, but there are ways that you can contribute to the development of your spiritual health.

Firstly, you could introduce meditation into a routine. This allows you to spend time in active spiritual practice. Whether you spend this time immersing yourself in nature, or whether you use this time to spend time with and bond with your creator, you will find your spiritual self-thanking you for it.

If you are also new to meditation techniques, there are many that you could pursue. Meditation could be sitting in absolute silence, allowing your mind to think about the magnificence of the world we live in or the magnificence of your creator. It can be through the practice of yoga which plays an active role in helping individuals reach spiritual enlightenment. You could use chants to find this spiritual health, or you could actively use prayer, attending religious services, and other spiritually specific practices of the belief system to follow to help you on your spiritual journey.

Much like health, spirituality is something you constantly pursue. You are never at a point in your life where you are at the height of your spirituality. Something will happen that may cause you to feel like you are slipping away from your spirituality, and the great thing about that is that you can humble yourself once more and begin your journey all over again.

Once you have found this holistic balance in your life, you will find yourself being one with your physical, mental, and spiritual self. You will feel whole and complete, and you can continue working toward maintaining this feeling.

Chapter 12:

Final Thoughts and Takeaways

We are all about fitness, we are all about the beauty that a healthier lifestyle will bring to us. Remember, the reason why we are pursuing health. I lost my dad to things in his life that could have been mitigated if he had taken better care of his health. When I lost him, all I kept thinking was how I would never want my kids to face the hurt and heartbreak of losing a parent in this same way. The reality is that our health and our longevity lie in our own hands. Yes, we could wake up tomorrow and be in a car crash. But I made a promise to myself that I would never allow my children to deal with the consequences of losing me prematurely because I never took care of my health.

I know, this seems extremely morbid, but that is the truth. And when you find a motivation strong enough to get you through the temptation and the falls, you will always find a reason to get back up all over again. The challenges will always present themselves. You just need to make sure that you are able to overcome the challenges when they inevitably present themselves.

As wonderful and magnificent as it is to pursue health and weight loss in a way that would work for most people, it is important to consult with a physician and a nutritionist before you pursue any form of diet, eating plan, or exercise program. If, for any reason, you cannot pursue your weight loss journey in the generic sense of the word, it is not the end of the road. You are not at a point where you have to expect an unhealthy lifestyle. All it means is finding a different way of pursuing this weight loss and health journey. It means working toward your own personal health that doesn't fit a one size fits all approach. And that's ok. The fact that you are putting the effort in already means that you are halfway there.

Once you learn what your limits are, you can make sure that you don't do anything to push those limits too far. Before you know it, you may even overcome the limits that once existed. You may be in a position that entirely eradicates the very things that once stood in your way. But for now, you start small and work within your limitations. Make yourself stronger and you'll be surprised at what you can do.

Common Weight Loss Mistakes

Weight loss is not something new. The pursuit of health is not something new. Because this has been around for hundreds of years, mistakes and flaws in the systems have been identified. They have been figured out and this information has been made available for people all around the world to make the right decisions and choices in their weight loss journey.

The first mistake that many women make is focusing solely on the number on the scale. The scale is such an unreliable tool for weight management and when you consider that weight can fluctuate at different times of the day or that water can make you weigh far more, it can be easy to throw you off and make you think you are far worse off than you actually are. If you really want to monitor your progress, the better way to do so would be to take your body measurements with a tape measure. But still, focusing too much on numbers is not good. Instead, the true test of health is how good you feel. Progress will eventually show, but it will now show if you are on the scale every day.

If you are someone who goes on the scale every day or who measures their body every day, stop and ask yourself what you are expecting. Are you expecting to see major changes in weight loss? Are you expecting to see weight gain? Are you expecting it to be the same number you saw it was yesterday? The reason why you are going on the scale every day is that you have some form of expectation. Whatever that expectation means you are either going to be happy or sad by the result you see. When you confront these expectations, you allow yourself to answer to yourself and you can make yourself realize that whatever result it is that you are hoping for, you are not going to see it in one day.

The next mistake that people make is that they either overeat or undereat. You see, many people don't realize how many calories they are actually eating because they don't check the labels. Let me put this into perspective for you. How many times have you decided that you are going to go for the healthier choice, and you are going to eat a salad at lunch instead of a steak? It was a beautiful salad, a bit flavorless, but that's alright because you drizzled some olive oil over it, and not to mention, you felt great afterward. But what you don't realize is that that one tablespoon of olive oil that you drizzled all over your salad added an extra 120 calories to your salad. To make matters worse, you thought that you did so well that day, you definitely ate the right amount of calories and so you rewarded yourself with a pizza. The reality is that it wasn't about how much or how little you ate, the reality is that you didn't know how to count your calories correctly and that is why you were eating salads which felt like nothing. You felt like you were starving, but you were gaining weight, or you just weren't losing weight.

Just like the mistake people make with food, they make the same mistake with exercising where they find themselves over or under-exercising. You may sit and wonder if you can go too far in either direction when it comes to eating because ultimately, you want to exercise for your health as well. But sometimes, we overdo it, and we jeopardize our entire weight loss journey because we get injured, we are unable to exercise, we find ourselves falling back into old and bad habits, and this leads us to gaining weight and slipping into depression because we allow ourselves to end up in this situation.

You may think that this example is exaggerated, but you don't know how deep and dark the black hole of misery is until you've fallen down and somehow managed to pick yourself up. Remember, too much of a good thing can be bad for you, so make sure that you know your limits.

One of the most common weight loss mistakes that women tend to make, is one that has already been mentioned in this book. But the reality is that it happens so often it needs to be mentioned again. Some women are of the firm belief that they tend to only do cardio to lose weight and that they shouldn't do any weight training to lose weight. This is a big mistake because muscle is needed to lose weight. They neglect to train the very thing that helps them lose weight faster. So, this is my advice to you—don't neglect weight and strength training. Lift weights and you will find that it does a lot of good for you.

Yes, we constantly talk about a calorie deficit, but how do you know if you are in a deficit? In order to know how many calories you can consume to lose weight, you need to know how much you burn during the day. Many people make the mistake of overestimating just how much they burn in the day. It is always worth it to have it calculated by a professional and figure out your calorie intake and expenditure. This will make your weight loss journey much better.

In the pursuit of major weight loss, many people find themselves focusing too much on eating salads, and they don't focus on what the body needs, which is protein and fiber. When you are venturing down your path to weight loss, remember that you are striving for balance. You need a little bit of everything to make sure you come out healthier on the other end and not deficient in anything.

Weight loss and health is hard, but it is oh-so-worth it. When you know what you need and you have the knowledge behind your pursuits, your journey doesn't become easier, but it has fewer bumps in the road.

Conclusion

There are so many elements that need to be considered in weight loss. If it was simple, 38.9% of the world wouldn't be obese (Elflein, 2022). But what the world doesn't know is that even though it is hard, if you implement certain aspects into your lifestyle, they become second nature and you will be able to live a healthier and more fulfilling lifestyle.

In this book, we have seen the importance of mental health, willpower, and mental strength; we have seen how important it is to eat correctly and exercise; we have learned how each person's body type will ultimately impact how successful their weight loss journey is and how the weight loss programs they ultimately pursue needs to be tailor-made for their body type. We have seen that psychology plays a monumental role in weight loss and overall health, and we have seen that without goals, you won't get very far in your weight loss journey.

What many people fail to realize is that none of the above things happens without the other. You need to find your place of health, but it usually comes with aches, discomfort, and adjustments to a new normal that you will ultimately create for yourself. And why do we do this? Well, that's the most important part, isn't it? Without a good enough *why*, you have no reason to change the life you are currently living.

You need to find your reason and your motivation. It needs to be a motivation that will weather the storm of temptation and that will serve as a pillar of strength and stability when the going gets tough... and trust me, it will get tough. When you have the motivation to overcome all the setbacks and drawbacks, you will be able to effortlessly pick yourself back up and get back on the horse.

If you can't find motivation in someone else, where better to start than in yourself? The fact that you are here, at the end of this book means that you want a healthy lifestyle enough to actively pursue it. You have put in the effort to find and read this book, now; it is time to take the theory and put it into practice.

Remember that unrealistic expectations and time limits are the enemies of your success. You determine your own health, so don't become your own enemy.

I am someone who has been at the very bottom; I have been at the lowest I have ever been, having unhealthy eating habits, living a life I despised, and not liking the person I saw in the mirror very much. But you know what is the best thing about being at your lowest? You can only go upwards from there!

Now that you have all the tools you need, go out there, use them, and become the best version of yourself that you can be!

References

Ayuda, T. (2020, October 12). *11 best exercises for weight loss in 2020, according to experts.* Prevention. https://www.prevention.com/weight-loss/a20474562/best-weight-loss-exercises/

Benefiber. (n.d.). *Why high fiber guts are good for gut health.* Www.benefiber.com. https://www.benefiber.com/amp/how-fiber-improves-gut-health.html

Boogaard, K. (2021, December 26). *Write achievable goals with the SMART goals framework. Work Life by Atlassian;* Atlassian. https://www.atlassian.com/blog/productivity/how-to-write-smart-goals

Bowers, E. S. (2012). *Weight management tips for people with depression - major depression center - everyday health.* EverydayHealth. https://www.everydayhealth.com/hs/major-depression/weight-management-for-depression/

Bushman, B. (2017, May 15). *7 ways to overcome depression without medication.* Intermountain Healthcare. https://intermountainhealthcare.org/blogs/topics/live-well/2017/05/7-ways-to-overcome-depression-without-medication/

CDC. (2020a, May 19). *Body mass index (BMI).* Centers for Disease Control and Prevention. https://www.cdc.gov/healthyweight/assessing/bmi/index.html#:~:text=Body%20Mass%20Index%20(BMI)%20is

CDC. (2020b, October 28). *Physical activity for a healthy weight.* Centers for Disease Control and Prevention.

https://www.cdc.gov/healthyweight/physical_activity/index.ht
ml

CDC. (2021). *Tips for coping with stress*. CDC. https://www.cdc.gov/violenceprevention/about/copingwith-stresstips.html

Centers for Disease Control and Prevention. (2019). *Assessing your weight*. Centers for Disease Control and Prevention. https://www.cdc.gov/healthyweight/assessing/index.html

Clear, J. (2012, December 10). *The beginner's guide to intermittent fasting*. James Clear. https://jamesclear.com/the-beginners-guide-to-intermittent-fasting

Cleveland Clinic. (2021). *Body contouring: What is it, benefits, risks & recovery*. Cleveland Clinic. https://my.clevelandclinic.org/health/treatments/21525-body-countouring

Davis, K. (2019, January 15). *Successful weight loss: 10 tips to lose weight*. Www.medicalnewstoday.com. https://www.medicalnewstoday.com/articles/303409

Decathlon Blog. (2022). *Healthy weight loss diet plan for female (diet chart included)*. Decathlon Blog. https://blog.decathlon.in/articles/weight-loss-indian-diet-chart

Eat Right. (2018). *Back to basics for healthy weight loss*. Eat Right. https://www.eatright.org/health/wellness/your-overall-health/back-to-basics-for-healthy-weight-loss

Elflein, J. (2022). *Topic: Obesity worldwide*. Statista. https://www.statista.com/topics/9037/obesity-worldwide/#:~:text=It%20is%20estimated%20that%20around%2038.9%20percent%20of%20the%20world

Felman, A. (2020, April 19). *Health: What does good health really mean?* MedicalNewsToday. https://www.medicalnewstoday.com/articles/150999#types

Fields, L. (2020, January 20). *5 ways to cultivate the power of positive thinking (and lose weight) | weight loss | myfitnesspal.* MyFitnessPal Blog. https://blog.myfitnesspal.com/5-ways-to-cultivate-the-power-of-positive-thinking-and-lose-weight/

Frey, M. (2021, June 28). *How to overcome 5 psychological blocks to weight loss.* Verywell Fit. https://www.verywellfit.com/overcome-emotional-stress-to-lose-weight-3495947

Ghosh, A. (2017, July 6). *10 scary side effects of over exercising.* Femina. https://www.femina.in/wellness/fitness/10-scary-side-effects-of-over-exercising-54707.html

Gunnars, K. (2019, July 3). *Top 12 biggest myths about weight loss.* Healthline. https://www.healthline.com/nutrition/top-12-biggest-myths-about-weight-loss#TOC_TITLE_HDR_2

Harvard T.H. Chan. (2018, March 27). *Diet review: Ketogenic diet for weight loss.* The Nutrition Source. https://www.hsph.harvard.edu/nutritionsource/healthy-weight/diet-reviews/ketogenic-diet/#:~:text=A%20decrease%20in%20appetite%2Dstimulating

Helfgott, M. (2022). *The importance of gut health.* Www.parkview.com. https://www.parkview.com/community/dashboard/the-importance-of-gut-health#:~:text=What%20is%20gut%20health%3F

Helmer, J. (2020, May 12). *Studies show: Your mindset affects the number on the scale | wellness | myfitnesspal.* MyFitnessPal Blog. https://blog.myfitnesspal.com/studies-show-your-mindset-affects-the-number-on-the-scale/

Hochwald, L., & Barrie, L. (2022). *21 tips for weight loss that actually work | everyday health.* EverydayHealth.com. https://www.everydayhealth.com/diet-and-nutrition/diet/tips-weight-loss-actually-work/

Holland, K. (2022, May 23). *22 ways to fight depression.* Healthline. https://www.healthline.com/health/depression/how-to-fight-depression#today-vs-tomorrow

Holmes Place. (2018, April 9). *7 daily habits to help you lose weight.* Holmes Place Corporate; Holmes Place. https://www.holmesplace.com/en/en/blog/lifestyle/7-daily-habits-to-help-you-lose-weight

Howley, E. K., & Fetters, K. A. (2022). *Ways to shift your mindset for better weight loss.* U.S. News. https://health.usnews.com/wellness/articles/ways-to-shift-your-mindset-for-better-weight-loss

Igo, C. (2022). *Keto diet: Everything you should know before you start.* CNET. https://www.cnet.com/health/how-to-go-keto-a-beginners-guide-to-the-keto-diet/

Institute for the Psychology of Eating. (2018). *The psychology of weight loss – psychology of eating.* Psychologyofeating.com. https://psychologyofeating.com/psychology-weight-loss/

Jang, H. J., Kim, B. S., Won, C. W., Kim, S. Y., & Seo, M. W. (2020). The relationship between psychological factors and weight gain. *Korean Journal of Family Medicine, 41*(6), 381–368. https://doi.org/10.4082/kjfm.19.0049

Johns Hopkins Medicine. (n.d.). *Intermittent fasting: What is it, and how does it work?* Www.hopkinsmedicine.org. https://www.hopkinsmedicine.org/health/wellness-and-prevention/intermittent-fasting-what-is-it-and-how-does-it-work#:~:text=What%20is%20intermittent%20fasting%3F

Leonard, J. (2018, June 28). *12 healthy high-fat foods.* Medical News Today. https://www.medicalnewstoday.com/articles/322295

Lino, C. (2016, October 2). *What is willpower? The psychology behind self-control.* PositivePsychology. https://positivepsychology.com/psychology-of-willpower/#:~:text=Researchers%20on%20self%2Dcontrol%20also

Livingston, M. (2021). *The best exercises for losing weight, according to fitness pros.* CNET. https://www.cnet.com/health/fitness/these-are-the-best-types-of-workouts-for-weight-loss/

M&S Team. (2018, July 10). *Muscle & strength's 10 week women's fat loss workout.* Muscle & Strength. https://www.muscleandstrength.com/workouts/muscle-and-strength-womens-fat-loss-workout

Medline Plus. (2018). *Are you getting too much exercise?: MedlinePlus medical encyclopedia.* Medlineplus. https://medlineplus.gov/ency/patientinstructions/000807.htm

Migala, J. (2020, January 6). *Body type diet: Are you an ectomorph, mesomorph, or endomorph? | everyday health.* EverydayHealth. https://www.everydayhealth.com/diet-nutrition/body-type-diet-are-you-ectomorph-mesomorph-endomorph/

Milkman, K. (2021, November 29). *How to build a habit in 5 steps, according to science.* CNN. https://edition.cnn.com/2021/11/29/health/5-steps-habit-builder-wellness/index.html

National Health Service. (2019, July 15). *What is the body mass index (BMI)? NHS;* NHS. https://www.nhs.uk/common-health-questions/lifestyle/what-is-the-body-mass-index-bmi/

NHS. (2021a, October 28). *12 tips to help you lose weight.* Nhs.uk. https://www.nhs.uk/live-well/healthy-weight/managing-your-weight/12-tips-to-help-you-lose-weight/

NHS. (2021b, November 25). *10 weight loss myths.* NHS. https://www.nhs.uk/live-well/healthy-weight/managing-your-weight/ten-weight-loss-myths/

Petre, A. (2020, December 14). *How to meal prep — A beginner's guide.* Healthline. https://www.healthline.com/nutrition/how-to-meal-prep#methods

Ratini, M. (2022). *10 diet mistakes and how to avoid them.* WebMD. https://www.webmd.com/diet/ss/slideshow-diet-mistakes

Riopel, L. (2019, June 14). *The importance, benefits, and value of goal setting.* PositivePsychology. https://positivepsychology.com/benefits-goal-setting/#:~:text=Setting%20goals%20helps%20trigger%20new

Saleh, N. (2020, March 19). *9 adverse health effects of too much exercise.* MDLinx. https://www.mdlinx.com/article/9-adverse-health-effects-of-too-much-exercise/70VZzE7JPAtHBOXq4O8Ltw

Schemper, A. (2022, August 13). *What does "toning" really mean?* Bodyfit by Amy. https://bodyfitbyamy.com/2022/08/13/what-does-toning-really-mean/

Scher, B. (2019, April 25). *Diet doctor.* Diet Doctor. https://www.dietdoctor.com/intermittent-fasting

Scott, E. (2019). *How stress can cause weight gain.* Verywell Mind. https://www.verywellmind.com/how-stress-can-cause-weight-gain-3145088

Stachel, J. (2022). *7 signs of a healthy gut + tips to improve digestive health - blog | everlywell: Home health testing made easy.* Everlywell. https://www.everlywell.com/blog/food-allergy/signs-of-healthy-gut/

Sutin, A. R. (2022). *Psychosocial dynamics of body weight.* APA. https://www.apa.org/science/about/psa/2014/09/body-weight#:~:text=Early%20investigations%20into%20the%20association

The Healthline Editorial Team. (2018). *Keto diet side effects.* Healthline. https://www.healthline.com/health-news/worst-side-effects-of-the-keto-diet

Tracy, B. (2019, September 6). *Importance of goal setting: 6 reasons to take setting goals seriously.* Brian Tracy International.

https://www.briantracy.com/blog/personal-success/goal-setting/

UCI Health. (2020). *The psychology behind maintaining weight loss.* Www.ucihealth.org. https://www.ucihealth.org/blog/2020/01/weight-loss-psychology

Vasile, C. (2020). Mental health and immunity (review). *Experimental and Therapeutic Medicine,* *20*(6), 1–1. https://doi.org/10.3892/etm.2020.9341

Weight Matters. (n.d.). *Psychological factors in obesity.* WeightMatters. https://weightmatters.co.uk/disordered-eating/psychological-factors-in-obesity/

Wellnessed. (2011, November 2). *The 3 body types: Ectomorph, mesomorph & endomorph.* Wellnessed. https://wellnessed.com/body-types/#:~:text=There%20are%203%20main%20body

Zelman, K. M. (n.d.). *The abcs of weight loss.* WebMD. https://www.webmd.com/fitness-exercise/features/the-abcs-of-weight-loss

Zelman, K. M. (2007). *8 ways to think thin.* WebMD. https://www.webmd.com/diet/obesity/features/8-ways-to-think-thin

Printed in Great Britain
by Amazon

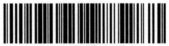

18317759R00068